the fast
800
recipe book

the fast 800 recipe book

Low-carb, Mediterranean-style recipes
for intermittent fasting and long-term health

DR CLARE BAILEY
and JUSTINE PATTISON

Foreword by DR MICHAEL MOSLEY

Published in 2019 by
Short Books,
Unit 316, ScreenWorks,
22 Highbury Grove,
London, N5 2ER

10 9 8 7 6 5 4 3 2 1

A CIP catalogue record for this book is available from the British Library.

ISBN: 978-1-78072-4133

Recipe consultant: Justine Pattison
Recipe testers: Claire Bignell, Karen Brooks, Jess Blain
Nutritional analysis: Fiona Hunter
Project editor: Jo Roberts-Miller
Design and art direction: Smith & Gilmour
Photography: Smith & Gilmour
Food styling: Phil Mundy
Props styling: Olivia Wardle
Cover design: Smith & Gilmour

Printed at CPI Colour Ltd, Croydon, CR0 4TD

FSC
www.fsc.org
MIX
Paper from
responsible sources
FSC® C016486

Contents

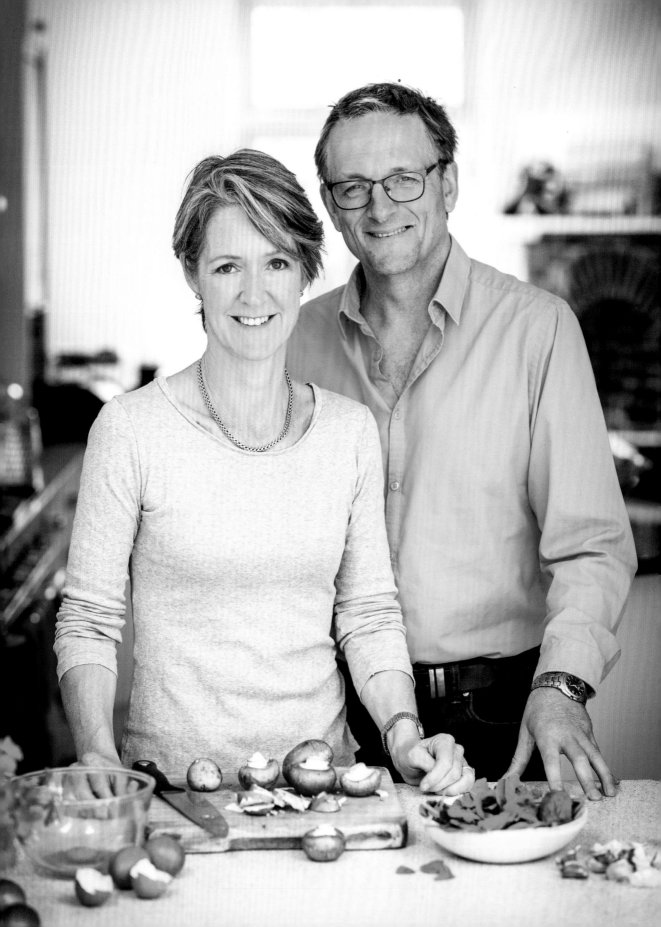

Foreword by Michael Mosley

It was in 2012 that I discovered, thanks to a random blood test, that I was a Type 2 diabetic. Rather than start on medication, I researched the benefits of intermittent fasting and started on what I called The 5:2 Diet, cutting my calories for two days a week and eating normally for the other five. I lost 9kg (nearly 20lb) and returned my blood sugars to normal.

Since then there has been a revolution in our understanding of the benefits of rapid weight loss. In fact, NHS Choices, which once described the 5:2 as a 'fad diet', now says that, 'Sticking to a regimen for two days a week can be more achievable than seven days, so you may be more likely to persevere with this way of eating and successfully lose weight. Two days a week on a restricted diet can lead to greater reductions in body fat, insulin resistance and other chronic diseases.'

Based on the latest science, I recently wrote a new book, *The Fast 800*, which pulls together everything I've learned about the easiest and most effective ways to lose weight and keep it off. In that book I made some changes to the original 5:2, upping the number of calories I recommend you eat on a fasting day to 800, which is enough to ensure you get all the nutrients you need without going hungry, and introducing a rapid weight loss option (where you eat 800 calories a day, every day) in order to kickstart your diet, and reap many other health benefits, too. As in previous books, the recipes in *The Fast 800* were created by my wife, Dr Clare Bailey.

The Fast 800 rapidly became an international bestseller, bought and read by hundreds of thousands of people. There was immediate demand for a follow-up recipe book, which Clare, with the help of the acclaimed cook and food writer Justine Pattison, has duly delivered. Having tasted the recipes in this book, I can assure you they are both delicious and filling!

So why should you follow the Fast 800 programme? One of the main benefits of doing this diet is that you lose fat – fast – which is very motivating. Contrary to what we are often told, losing weight fast doesn't mean you will put it back on again, even faster.

A recent, hugely impressive study called DIRECT, carried out by Professors Mike Lean and Roy Taylor, showed that people with Type 2 diabetes who were randomly allocated an 800-calorie diet managed to lose and keep off far more weight than those who we were put on a slow and steady diet. Those allocated the 800-calorie regime lost an average of 10kg, which they kept off for more than a year, compared to just 1kg in the control group. Almost half were able to put their diabetes into remission (they got their blood sugars back to normal, despite not being on medication), compared to 4% in the control group.

Even more impressive was the follow-up study, which looked at what happened to those same patients two years later. Although there was some weight re-gain, the majority of those who had gone into remission were still in remission. And compared to the control group, they were far better off. Not only were they slimmer and with lower blood sugar levels, but they had lower cholesterol levels, lower blood pressure and were on far less medication. There were also far fewer serious side effects, such as heart attacks or new cases of cancer.

As Professor Lean said to me, 'For years we have been telling patients with Type 2 diabetes to take the pills and not worry too much. It is time to be honest and tell them that this is a serious disease with nasty complications, particularly if you develop it in your 40s or 50s. The good news is that with the right help many people can now get shot of it.'

I do hope you enjoy this book, a winning combination of art and science!

Introduction

Two of the great passions of my life have been food and medicine. Both my parents were doctors and my mother, who was a superb cook as well as a renowned child psychiatrist, taught me the joys of experimenting with food and combining flavours in different ways. She was also a believer in the impact of good food on mental health.

Following in her footsteps, I trained as a doctor at the Royal Free Hospital in London, where I met my husband, Michael Mosley, who has surprised me by going on to become a television presenter and health guru!

What surprises me even more, at least in retrospect, is how little we learned during our years at medical school and my subsequent GP training, about the impact of diet or exercise on health. We were aware of the importance of 'lifestyle advice' but most of the time we did what we were trained to do – prescribe medication, and in increasing quantities.

When I first qualified, in the 1980s, the standard advice, rarely questioned, was to tell patients to go on a 'low-fat diet'. The fact that this steered them towards eating more carbs, usually in the form of sweet, starchy and often highly processed foods, didn't seem to matter. After all, everyone 'knew' that the only real way to get fat was by eating fat. As we now know, that advice was not just unhelpful, it was wrong. Eating fat does not necessarily make you fat; and sticking to a low-fat diet can mean you are missing out on healthy natural fats, which not only make food taste better and keep you feeling full for longer, but provide important nutrients and vitamins.

When Michael discovered he had Type 2 diabetes it was a wake-up call. He managed to reverse his condition by losing a lot of weight fast on the 5:2 diet, and from then on, we both obsessively studied the evolving new science about the impact of food on health. Over the past seven years, new research has led to major developments in our understanding of the best ways to achieve weight loss, as well as life-changing advances in the prevention and reversal of diabetes.

I have recently been involved myself with an Oxford University study, 'The Dietary Approaches to the Management of Type 2 Diabetes (DIAMOND)', which put participants with Type 2 diabetes on a low-carb diet and an 8-week programme of 800cals a day, followed by 4 weeks of weight maintenance – the results of which look very promising. The message is now clear, Type 2 can be improved and even reversed by losing weight fast on a low-calorie or intermittent fasting diet.

In *The Fast 800* Michael has brought together all the latest scientific research to provide one highly flexible, easy-to-follow programme – aimed not just at diabetics and prediabetics, but anyone who wants to lose weight and keep it off. And this companion recipe book is designed to help you put that programme into practice, whatever your needs or goals. You may have a lot of weight to lose, you may have a medical condition that is improved by weight loss, you may only need to shift a bit of weight and want the flexibility of intermittent fasting, or perhaps you simply want the long-term benefits of maintaining this way of life.

I am delighted to have worked on this book with expert cook and food writer Justine Pattison. Together, we have created a collection of delicious recipes, which all follow the principles of a lowish-carb Mediterranean-style diet. These recipes are also tailored to support your microbiome – enabling those trillions of microbes living in your intestine to work more effectively on your behalf and produce substances that can boost your overall health and well-being, and even improve your mood.

There are numerous calorie-counted meals for you to choose from for your 800cals fast days, as well as tips for adapting them for non-fast days, when you are not calorie counting. You will also find a good selection of meal-replacement shakes, as much of the research on rapid weight loss has been done using these, and we have had many people inquiring about including them within the programme.

For me, as a GP, this has been an incredibly rewarding and exciting time. Sharing diet and lifestyle advice with patients has at last felt like pushing on an open door. At the same time, there has been a grass-roots surge of interest in intermittent fasting and uptake internationally, which has motivated thousands of people around the world to transform their lives and future health.

Many of my patients have told me that they love the flexibility of the Fast 800, with its combination of more manageable fasting days and lowish-carb Mediterranean-style food. They say it is the first diet they have been able to stick to and they are genuinely surprised that they no longer feel hungry all the time.

I do hope you like these recipes and that they help you to lose weight, while enjoying the food and feeling satiated. Finding a sustainable way of not just losing weight but keeping it off – that is the key to taking back control of your health.

DR CLARE BAILEY

A note from Justine Pattison

When Clare rang and asked me to help assemble the recipes for this book I was thrilled. I felt that my experience of writing cookbooks about weight loss and creating health-related recipes, combined with Clare and Michael's medical background and extensive knowledge about the impact of food on health, would make us a perfect fit.

To see how doable the diet really is, I tested the Fast 800 principles on myself. After indulging for a few weeks on lots of foods packed with starchy carbs, I embarked on the Fast 800 for four weeks, eating around 800cals a day. I rapidly lost 12 pounds and my energy levels soared. Despite a punishing work schedule, my skin glowed and I felt great. This also gave me great insight into how to tailor the recipes.

Clare and I have created recipes to fit into everyday life – simple to cook, using ingredients that are easily accessible and that taste delicious! Every recipe has been tested in my test kitchen. You'll find a wide variety here and we've added lots of extra tips and ideas for serving suggestions, using up leftovers and ideas about what to eat on non-fast days, too.

At the back of the book are handy meal plans to follow should you wish: two weeks of 800cals menus offering three meals a day; and two weeks of 800cals menus offering two meals a day, for those following a Time Restricted Eating (TRE) plan. And if you prefer to eat meat-free, there are also separate vegetarian meal plans.

Working with Clare on this book has been a huge pleasure and I hope you enjoy all the recipes as much as we do.

What is the Fast 800?

This diet is designed to be as flexible as possible, while incorporating the best science-based advice. All the meals are based on a lowish-carb Mediterranean-style way of eating, but how you manage the 800cals days is down to you.

Most people choose to kickstart their diet with a fast-track plan of 800cals a day, every day, for two or more weeks. They then move on to the New 5:2, cutting their calories for two days a week, and on the other days continuing to eat a healthy, Med-style diet, keeping carbohydrate intake low and controlling portion size. But you can tailor your regime to suit your needs. If you find the idea of the fast-track plan daunting, you could go straight to the New 5:2 and stick with that, in which case you will lose weight but not quite so quickly.

As Michael describes in his book, you can also add in a relatively new form of intermittent fasting called Time Restricted Eating (TRE), whereby you eat all your calories within a narrower time window each day – usually within 8 to 12 hours. This extends the length of your normal overnight fast (when you are sleeping and not eating) and gives your body an opportunity to burn fat and do essential repairs (see opposite for more information).

As with any diet, the Fast 800 may not suit everyone, so check with your health professional first (see page 12 for exclusions and cautions).

The Mediterranean-style makeover

While 'lowish' in carbohydrates, this is not a seriously restrictive diet, where you have to give up everything that contains carbs. However, it does mean reducing, and ideally avoiding, sugary foods. It also means cutting right back on starchy carbs, such as white bread, white pasta, rice and potatoes, as well as most breakfast cereals, since these readily convert to sugars in your body.

As a general principle, the Mediterranean-style way of eating involves moving away from processed foods and towards eating food cooked from scratch and prepared in a more traditional way – although, mindful of our time-poor lives, we have tried to keep the recipes as simple as possible.

The great thing about eating a Med-style diet, rather than a low-fat one, is that you can enjoy plenty of olive oil, avocados, some full-fat dairy, lots of nuts, seeds and oily fish – all the kinds of ingredients that make food tasty and filling. The programme also includes masses of vegetables, some fruit, as well as wholegrains, beans and lentils for extra fibre.

Rapid weight loss with 800-calorie fasting

We recommend that you start with this intensive stage, if possible. By sticking to 800cals a day, every day, for at least two weeks, you will kickstart your weight loss and better metabolic health. 800cals a day is low enough to induce mild ketosis, which is associated with fat burning, but high enough to ensure you get the nutrients you need.

After two weeks, pause and reflect on how it is going. If you are feeling good, losing weight and not struggling to stick to the diet, then carry on. You can continue this approach until you reach your goal or for up to 12 weeks.

Rapid weight loss is motivating and it is particularly helpful for people with a lot of weight to lose, for those with central obesity (excessive abdominal fat around the stomach) or who have raised blood sugars.

Some people find it helpful during this stage to make up some of their meals as shakes. See pages 50–53 for recipes or visit thefast800.com where we have developed ready-made meal replacement shakes with a Med-style formulation to help fill the gap.

STAGE 2

Intermittent fasting with the New 5:2

When you are nearing your target, or if you don't have much weight to lose, you can switch to the New 5:2. This is probably one of the easiest and most effective ways to lose weight and keep it off. We now recommend that, instead of reducing your calories to only 500–600 calories, as in the original 5:2 Fast Diet, you stick to 800 calories on fast days, while continuing to eat the Med-style way on non-fast days, not calorie counting, but exercising portion control.

STAGE 3

The lowish-carb Med-style diet and maintenance programme

Once you've hit your goal and grown to love the Med-style approach, you are in the groove – the maintenance phase. Stick to the general principles, using the recipe amends we offer for non-fast days and throwing in the odd fast day, and you are set for life. Enjoy the occasional treat, but try to maintain a diet low in sugar and moderately low in starchy carbohydrates, to help prevent sugars creeping up or weight piling back on. Relax a bit, but not too much! If your weight increases or your new outfit starts to feel tight, you know what to do...

Adding in Time Restricted Eating (TRE)

TRE enhances the benefits of the Fast 800. If you stop eating by 8pm and don't start again till 8am, that is a 12-hour fast (i.e. a 12:12). Start with this, then build up to a 14-hour fast (which means eating within a 10-hour window, a 14:10). Many people find that eating in a shorter window during the day makes it easier to manage a fast day. But it is a good habit to get into on non-fast days, too. See pages 246–7 for our menu plans based around two meals rather than three.

Benefits of the Fast 800 approach

There is a well-demonstrated, sustainable benefit to health in eating a moderately low-carb, Med-style diet and in being comfortably within a normal weight. People do the Fast 800 for a range of reasons:

● **To lose fat, fast:** as Michael says, one of the main benefits of doing the Fast 800 and the New 5:2 is rapid, sustainable weight loss, and that, contrary to what we are often told, losing weight fast doesn't mean you will put it back on again, even faster.

● **For general health and to live longer,** as well as for the sense of well-being and increased energy it brings. A recent study which compared people doing 5:2 intermittent fasting with standard dieting found the intermittent dieters were much more efficient at clearing fat from their blood after being given a fatty meal. Being overweight or obese also puts you at risk of developing common cancers, such as breast and bowel cancer. Excess fat, particularly around the gut, sends signals to the rest of your body telling your cells to divide more frequently, and getting rid of belly fat is a good way to counter that.

● **For metabolic reasons,** such as improving blood sugars, reversing and preventing diabetes, reducing blood pressure, improving cholesterol and lipid profile, reversing non-alcoholic fatty liver disease (NAFLD), reducing risks of coronary artery disease and strokes, reducing the risk of dementia (known also as Type 3 diabetes), reversing polycystic ovary syndrome (PCOS), as well as improving the chance of conception in obesity and reducing the risk of diabetes in pregnancy.

● **To power up your brain:** people who've done the Fast 800 report greater energy and clarity when they cut out sweet and starchy foods and go into mild ketosis. Research is increasingly confirming the benefits of this approach for reducing cognitive decline and even for increasing the production of new brain cells.

● **To boost your mood and motivation:** not only is the Mediterranean diet good for the heart and waist, it is also a great way to reduce depression and anxiety. In fact, studies have shown that those who stick closest to a traditional Mediterranean diet have a 33 per cent lower risk of developing depression than those who don't. Conversely, eating a diet containing lots of junk or processed food leads to much higher rates of depression.

● **To help reduce inflammation in the body,** leading to improvements in conditions such as arthritis, asthma and psoriasis, as well as reducing the risk of some cancers.

> **SAFETY: Exclusions and cautions**
> This diet is not suitable for under-18s, or if you're breastfeeding, pregnant or undergoing fertility treatment. Do not do it if you are underweight or have an eating disorder. Discuss with your GP if you are on medication or if you have a medical condition, including diabetes, low or high blood pressure, retinopathy or epilepsy. Nor should you do this if you are frail, unwell or whilst doing endurance exercise. (For more detailed information see https://thefast800.com/faqs/)

Seven ways to go lowish carb, Med-style

1 Reduce sugars and starchy foods. Most people realise they should be eating less cake, sweets, biscuits and sweetened drinks, but those are just the tip of the iceberg. There are all sorts of other culprits that contain hidden sugars, such as fruit juices, instant oats, most processed and many pre-prepared foods, white pasta, rice and bread, as well as potatoes and sweet potatoes. These foods convert into sugar in your blood almost as quickly as the white stuff itself.

A cautionary word on fruit – although fresh fruit contains fibre and healthy nutrients, it also contains lots of sugar. (See overleaf for more on which fruits are best and when to eat them.)

2 Eat decent amounts of protein every day. Your body can't store protein. If deprived, it will break down your own protein and muscles to get what it needs. Aim for around 45–60g of protein most days, even on 800cals days. Include plenty of oily fish, seafood, chicken, eggs, some full-fat dairy, some red meat, as well as tofu, beans, lentils, Quorn and nuts. Restrict processed meats, such as bacon, sausages or salami, although we do include small quantities in some recipes for protein and flavour.

3 Increase your consumption of natural healthy fats, mainly plant-based. Being energy-dense, fat is an excellent slow-release form of energy that keeps you going without pushing up sugars. And many high-fat foods are extremely nutritious.

So, enjoy adding in lovely extra-virgin olive oil, and eating some full-fat dairy, ideally in fermented form, such as cheese and yoghurt, as well as satiating avocado, salmon and oily fish, and nuts and seeds. Avoid low-fat diet products and highly processed fats.

4 Fill half your plate with non-starchy veg, such as spinach, kale, chard, spring greens and cabbage, as well as green beans, peppers, courgettes, broccoli, cauliflower and salad leaves. All these vegetables contain lots of nutrients, as well as fibre that helps the 'good' microbes in your gut to thrive. In fact, these are so important that we have decided to release you from having to calorie count them! If you are not a fan, you might find that eating these vegetables cooked with extra seasoning, or with added flavours, converts you, particularly on a fast day – it is said that hunger is the best sauce! (See page 241 for ideas on how to add interest to your greens.)

5 Avoid snacking between meals, or late-night grazing. The trouble with snacking is that it reduces fat burning. If you must snack on a fast day, eat a small portion of non-starchy vegetables, such as sliced cucumber, broccoli or celery. We include some recipes for dips (see pages 106–7), but these are best eaten as part of a meal. Alternatively, try a few nuts (one portion is the amount that will sit on the palm of your hand) or a sliver of cheese.

6 Swap white rice and pasta for wholemeal versions and pulses, such as lentils, quinoa and beans. Best eaten in moderation, these 'complex carbohydrates' are a particularly good source of fibre – the ideal 'fertiliser' to keep your microbiome happy and healthy – and are key to the success of a Mediterranean diet, which is 'lowish' in carbs in contrast to a very low-carb diet where many high-fibre healthy carbs are avoided, too. We encourage you to add them in on non-fast days.

7 Drink healthily. It is vital, when you are reducing calories and losing weight, to make sure you remain well hydrated by adding extra fluids – mainly water, if you can. Otherwise, stick to black tea, fruit teas and black coffee (see page 244 for some suggestions for other no-cal drinks). Avoid anything with added calories. And any drinks containing sweeteners. Although it's best to avoid alcohol on 800cals days, you can enjoy the occasional glass of red wine on non-fast days in the spirit of the Mediterranean diet.

Q and A

How do I get started?
It takes time and effort to adjust to a new way of eating. And it is easy to get hung up on willpower – or one's apparent lack of it. So, the most important thing is good planning. It helps to write down why you want to do the diet and, specifically, what your goals are. Go out and tell people, too, as you are more likely to stick to it. Clear away tempting and unhealthy foods, if you can. And then, just set a day to start. The first few weeks are the toughest. But once your body has adapted to fat-burning, it gets easier and you should find that you feel a great deal better – more energetic, clearer-headed and less tired – which is highly motivating.

Should I drink more on my 800cals days?
Being dehydrated is the main reason people give up on fast days – it leaves you feeling feeble, light headed and with brain fog, symptoms often mistakenly attributed to being on a low-cal regime. When you cut back your calories, not only do you miss the usual fluid in food, you also lose water as part of the process of breaking down fat. So, drinking extra fluids can be key to success – most people will require 1–1.5 litres extra each day, particularly if it's hot or you are active.

Which oils are best?
As a rule of thumb, the less processed the oils the better. Cold-pressed oils, such as extra-virgin olive and rapeseed oil, are minimally processed, retaining their beneficial nutrients. But they are more expensive than more refined oils. For a cheaper alternative choose light olive oil. Peanut oil is good for making stir fries and we like to use coconut oil, especially in baking and some Asian foods. But olive oil is king. On non-fast days when you are not worrying about calorie-counting – and even on fast days, when you just need to be mindful of the extra calories – we would encourage you to be generous with it. It tastes gorgeous, keeps you full for longer and has plenty of health benefits. And don't worry about the 'smoke point' when frying, as olive oil has been found to be safe when heated at regular temperatures.

What kind of seasoning should I be using?
We use plenty of freshly ground black pepper and flaked sea salt, such as Maldon, as this gives more flavour with less salt due to finer crystals.

How much meat should I eat?
Michael and I are generally reducing the amount of meat we eat for health and environmental reasons. We have done this by stealth at home, so the kids haven't really noticed the change. And we are all thoroughly enjoying our meat-free meals. However, on a fasting day, eating meat is an effective way to ensure you get an adequate amount of protein. As for processed meats – only eat these occasionally and choose good-quality versions.

What about full-fat dairy?
As Michael explains in *The Fast 800*, it is time to dump the low-fat dairy products and go back to enjoying luscious, satiating, full-fat dairy, particularly the live fermented versions, such as Greek-style yoghurt, cheese or crème fraîche. Butter is back on the menu, too, in moderation, and is probably better for you than most processed spreads. For people who are dairy-free, there are plenty of good alternatives, such as unsweetened nut or oat milk – although you may need to factor in different calorie counts for these and they may be lower in protein (see page 240 for standard dairy calories).

Can I eat fruit?
Many of my patients graze on fruit throughout the day, making it the main part of their 5-a-day. Unfortunately, fruit is a natural sugar storage device, with tropical fruits, like pineapples, mangoes, bananas and watermelon, rating particularly highly. Snacking on these is likely to spike your blood sugars and stop fat-burning. Try and stick instead to berries and hard fruits, such as apples and pears, which also tend to be higher in fibre. Ideally, you should be eating them as part of a meal, rather than as a snack, and only two portions a day. Also, if you eat fruit when it is less ripe, the sugar content will be lower.

Is the Fast 800 suitable for vegetarians and/or vegans?
This diet is suitable for vegetarians and we have included vegetarian and meat-free recipes. To make it easier to get enough protein, we would recommend adding in extra where you can, such as a handful of nuts or seeds, portions of tofu, edamame, lentils, quinoa, peas or beans, even if this takes you up to 900cals on fast days – it's worth it. Adding high protein shakes can help. However, this diet is not specifically designed for vegans, who can find it more of a challenge to achieve adequate protein and nutrients while only eating 800cals. Making a fasting diet suitable for vegans requires careful planning, and is best done with professional support.

Should I take vitamins?
We recommend taking a good-quality multivitamin on 800cals fasting days, to make sure you get the vitamins and minerals you need.

How long is it safe to do the Fast 800?
Rapid weight loss for up to 12 weeks has been shown to be safe, and has been used in research. But stick to our recommendations and make sure you drink plenty of water. Some people continue for longer. However, we would recommend that once you reach your goal, or after three months, you start introducing non-fasting days each week. On these days you should practise portion control as part of a Med-style diet and move towards an intermittent fasting regime. (See Stage 2 on page 11.)

Should I tell my doctor/ health professional? It is always a good idea to keep them informed about a major change to your diet, particularly if you have a medical condition and/ or are on medication (see page 12 for exclusions and cautions). It may help to print out a letter advising them about the diet, so they can monitor and support you in the process. This can be found at thefast800.com. Most health professionals will be aware of this approach and will be supportive.

Tips for using this book

Calorie counts
All the calorie counts given on the recipes refer to one individual serving, unless stated otherwise. That said, please be aware that we include calorie counts as a rough guide only. There are variations between different nutritionists, counters and apps, and you should not be too concerned by a few extra calories here or there. In fact, we have made non-starchy vegetables, such as leafy greens, broccoli, salad leaves, radishes, runner beans and celery, into 'no counting' options, as the calories in these foods are insignificant compared with their nutritional benefits. If a recipe includes a serving suggestion, such as a salad or some steamed greens, these can be considered a free non-counting extra – unless you want to add a dressing or a teaspoonful of extra-virgin olive oil, in which case, see page 241 for calories.

Non-fast days
For those days when you are not sticking to 800cals – i.e. if you are on the New 5:2 or have moved on to the Maintenance stage – we offer suggestions and tips for how to adapt the recipes to make them more substantial. These might involve simply increasing or doubling the portion size, or adding a few tablespoons of brown rice or lentils, an extra glug of olive oil, a slice of seeded bread or extra vegetables.

Make the recipes suit you
These recipes are based on a Mediterranean-style way of eating, but can be adapted to fit different cuisines and tastes. Feel free to adjust them by using alternative flavours, or adding different herbs and spices – all of which have minimal impact on calories. You could turn a basic Bolognese into a spicy Mexican dish, or Mediterranean vegetables into a curry. The more tasty and satisfying your food, the more likely you are to stick to this way of eating.

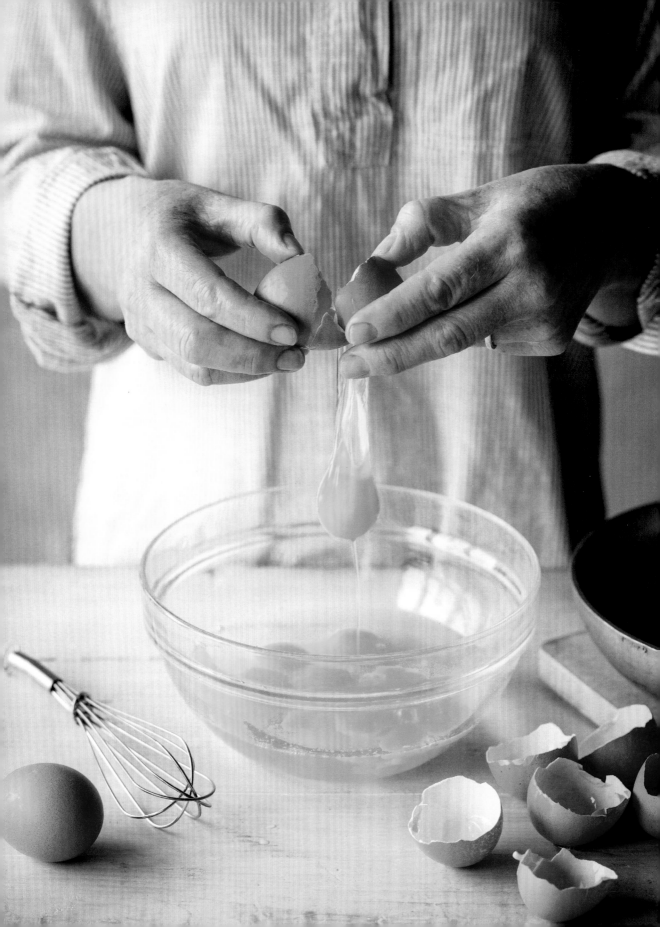

Breakfast and Brunch

Breakfast is often described as the most important meal of the day, but there are no hard and fast rules as to when you should eat it. Both Michael and I love breakfast, but if you prefer to skip it or eat it later, that's fine; and by doing so you are extending your overnight fast – an effective form of intermittent fasting called TRE (see pages 10–11). We include a variety of breakfast options, from quick and easy to relaxed brunches, and food to eat on the go. But, whether you eat anything or not, you MUST drink plenty of fluids to keep you going until you do 'break your fast'.

Pear and cinnamon porridge

SERVES 1

30g jumbo porridge oats
1 Conference pear (around
    135g), peeled, cored and
    roughly chopped
¼ tsp ground cinnamon
75ml full-fat milk
5g toasted flaked almonds
    (around 2 tsp)

NON-FAST DAYS
Increase the portion size.

A comforting and filling breakfast. You can substitute the pear with a grated apple, if you like.

1 Place the oats, pear and cinnamon into a small non-stick saucepan. Pour in the milk and 120ml water and cook over a low–medium heat for 5–6 minutes, stirring constantly, or until the oats are softened and creamy.

2 Pour into a deep bowl and scatter with the flaked almonds to serve.

COOK'S TIP

★ If you can't find ready-toasted almonds, toast your own in a dry frying pan over a low heat for 1–2 minutes, stirring regularly; or simply top with the untoasted kind.

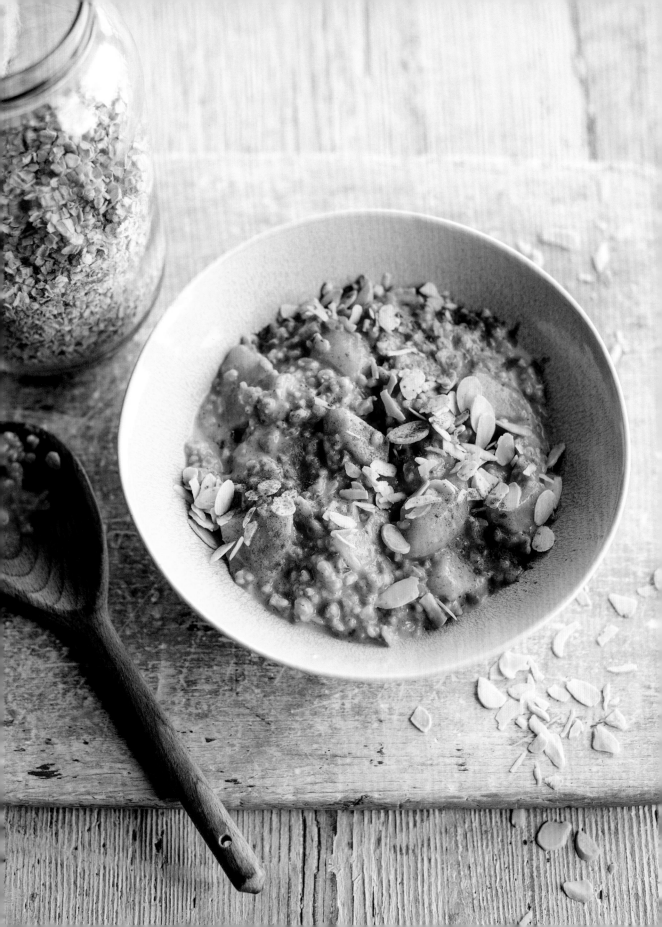

UNDER 300 CALORIES | PER SERVING | **274cals** | PROTEIN **8g** | FAT **16g** | FIBRE **3g** | CARBS **22g**

Chocolate granola

SERVES 8

4 tbsp coconut oil
1 tbsp cocoa powder
1 tbsp maple syrup
200g jumbo porridge oats
100g mixed nuts, roughly
    chopped
75ml full-fat milk
    (per serving)

NON-FAST DAYS
Add 100g finely chopped 85%
dark chocolate to the granola for
the last 5 minutes of the cooking
time. Don't stir but let it cool and
harden for a few hours before
putting it in the jar.

This easy breakfast is filling and full of fibre – a
wonderful alternative to sugary breakfast cereals.

1 Preheat the oven to 170°C/fan 150°C/Gas 3.

2 Melt the coconut oil with the cocoa powder and maple
syrup in a large non-stick saucepan over a gentle heat,
stirring regularly.

3 Remove from the heat and stir in the oats until
thoroughly coated. Scatter evenly over a baking tray
and bake for 15 minutes.

4 Remove from the oven and stir in the nuts. Return
to the oven for a further 10 minutes.

5 Remove from the oven and leave to cool and crisp
up on the tray.

6 Serve 40g granola with 75ml milk per person.

COOK'S TIPS

★ Store in an airtight jar for up to 2 weeks.
★ Serve with full-fat live Greek yoghurt instead, but
remember to adjust the calories. The 75ml full-fat milk
contains 47cals. Non-dairy milk can be used and the
calories calculated separately.
★ Buy your nuts ready mixed or chop your own selection.

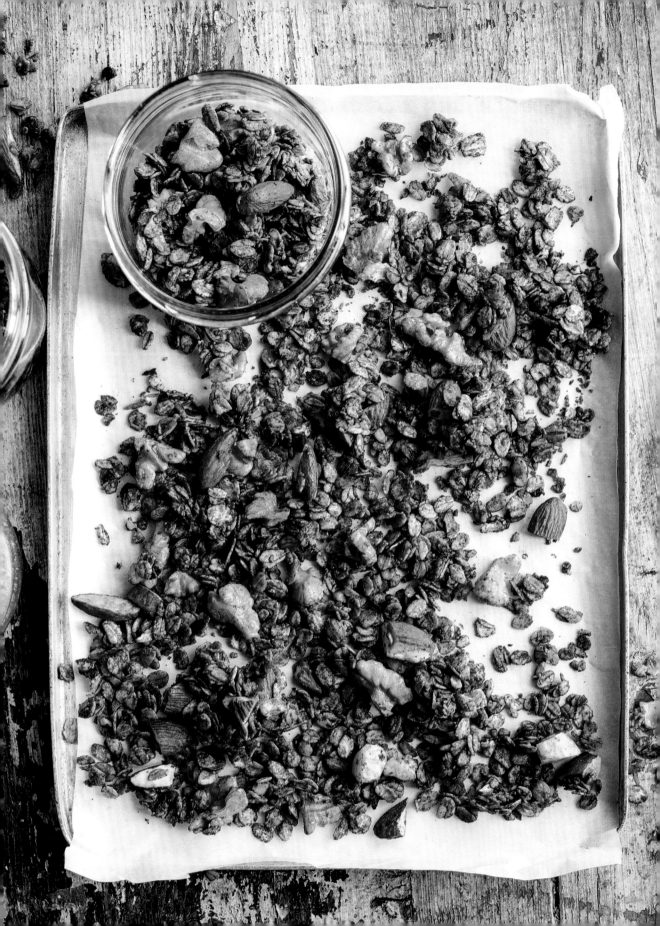

PER SERVING | **351cals** | PROTEIN **10.5g** | FAT **20g** | FIBRE **5.5g** | CARBS **30g**

Overnight oats

SERVES 2

1 small apple
60g jumbo porridge oats
25g toasted hazelnuts,
    roughly chopped
75g full-fat live Greek yoghurt
100ml full-fat milk
1 tbsp mixed seeds
50g blueberries or
    mixed berries

NON-FAST DAYS
Increase the portion size.

Soaking the oats in milk overnight softens them. The apple adds fibre and makes them extra juicy.

1 Coarsely grate the unpeeled apple, working your way carefully around the fruit, avoiding the core.

2 Put the grated apple into a bowl and stir in the oats, hazelnuts, yoghurt and milk. Cover and chill in the fridge for several hours or overnight.

3 Serve topped with the mixed seeds and berries.

COOK'S TIPS

★ You can use dairy-free yoghurt and milk for this recipe but you'll need to recalculate the calories accordingly. The 75g full-fat live Greek yoghurt contains 50cals and 100ml full-fat milk contains 63cals.
★ Store the overnight oats in small lidded containers to make this an easy portable breakfast, too.

Instant porridge in a cup

SERVES 1

40g porridge oats (not jumbo)
1 tbsp dried skimmed
  milk powder
8 walnut or pecan halves,
  roughly chopped

NON-FAST DAYS
Increase the portion size.

This very portable porridge is ideal if you're travelling or only have access to a kettle. Skimmed milk powder is easy to find in the supermarket and is often fortified for an extra vitamin boost.

1 Pour boiled water into a mug to heat it, then tip it away.

2 Place the oats and dried skimmed milk powder in the warmed mug and pour over just enough boiling water to cover – you'll need around 150ml. Stir well and put a plate over the top. Leave to stand for 3–5 minutes. Check the consistency and add extra water if needed. Stir again to release the starch and make the oats creamy.

3 Top with the nuts to serve.

COOK'S TIPS

★ This recipe uses plain porridge oats (rolled oats) rather than the chunkier jumbo kind, so they soften more easily.
★ Add ¼ teaspoon ground cinnamon to the dry ingredients if you like.
★ You could serve the porridge topped with a handful of fresh blueberries or a sliced banana, but remember to add the extra calories.

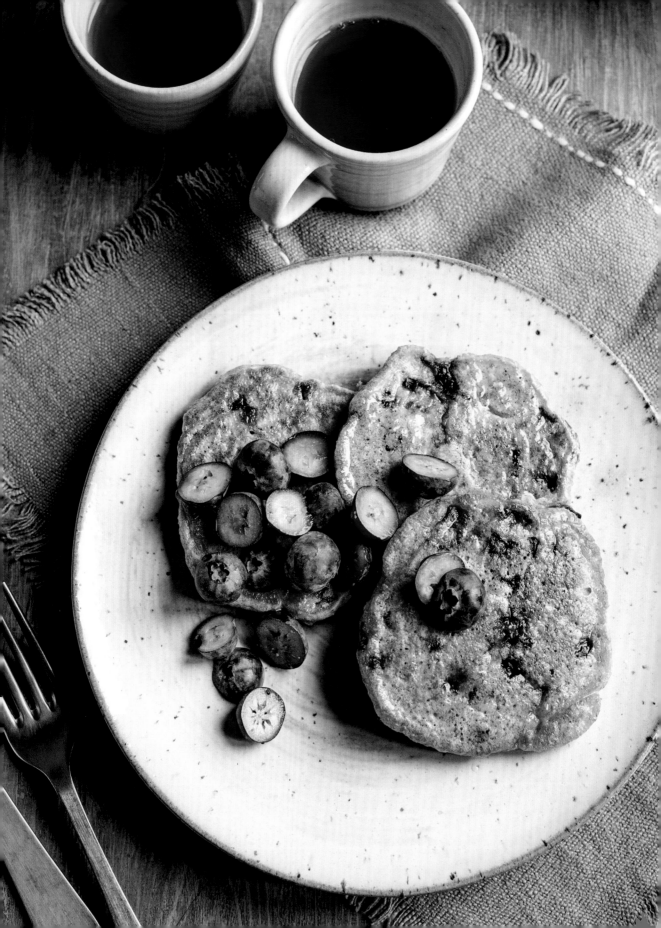

Blueberry pancakes

SERVES 2

**75g wholemeal
self-raising flour**
15g porridge oats (not jumbo)
1 large egg
100ml full-fat milk
125g blueberries
2 tsp rapeseed or coconut oil

NON-FAST DAYS
Top the pancakes with a
sliced banana or a handful
of fresh berries.

A weekend treat, which can be multiplied to serve
all the family. Use rolled porridge oats rather than
the jumbo variety for the best results.

1 Place the flour and oats in a bowl, make a well in the
centre and break the egg into it. Pour in half the milk and,
using a whisk, beat everything together to form a thick
batter. Add the remaining milk and beat hard until the
batter is smooth.

2 Tip the blueberries into a separate bowl, keeping some
aside for garnishing later, and lightly crush with the back
of a spoon before adding to the batter and mixing well.

3 Brush a large non-stick frying pan with a little of the
oil and place over a medium–high heat. Spoon a sixth of
the batter in a loose heap on one side of the pan and allow
to spread gently. Add two more spoonfuls in the same way.
Cook for 2 minutes, or until small bubbles appear on the
surface and the top is beginning to set, then carefully flip
over and cook on the other side for 1½–2 minutes.

4 Transfer the pancakes to a warmed plate and cook the
remaining three pancakes in the same way. Serve with
the reserved blueberries.

COOK'S TIPS

★ Use non-dairy milk if you prefer but remember to
adjust the calories. 100ml full-fat milk contains 63cals.
★ If you are making this breakfast for one, keep the
remaining pancakes for the next day. Reheat on a covered
plate in the microwave on high for around 30 seconds,
or until hot throughout.

Warm berry compote with yoghurt

SERVES 2

100g mixed frozen berries, any variety

2 soft pitted dates, finely chopped

200g full-fat live Greek yoghurt

NON-FAST DAYS
Sprinkle with toasted jumbo oats, mixed seeds or roughly chopped nuts.

A luscious combination that makes the most of frozen fruit. Choose a berry selection that includes naturally sweet strawberries or cherries if you can.

1 Put the frozen berries and dates in a small saucepan and heat gently for 3–5 minutes, or until the fruit has thawed and warmed, stirring regularly. Add a splash of water if needed, to help the fruit soften.

2 Divide the yoghurt between two bowls and spoon the warm compote on top. Eat immediately.

COOK'S TIPS

★ For a thicker compote, cook the fruit with 1 teaspoon chia seeds and a few extra tablespoons of water.

★ You could leave the compote to cool and serve with the yoghurt as a dessert.

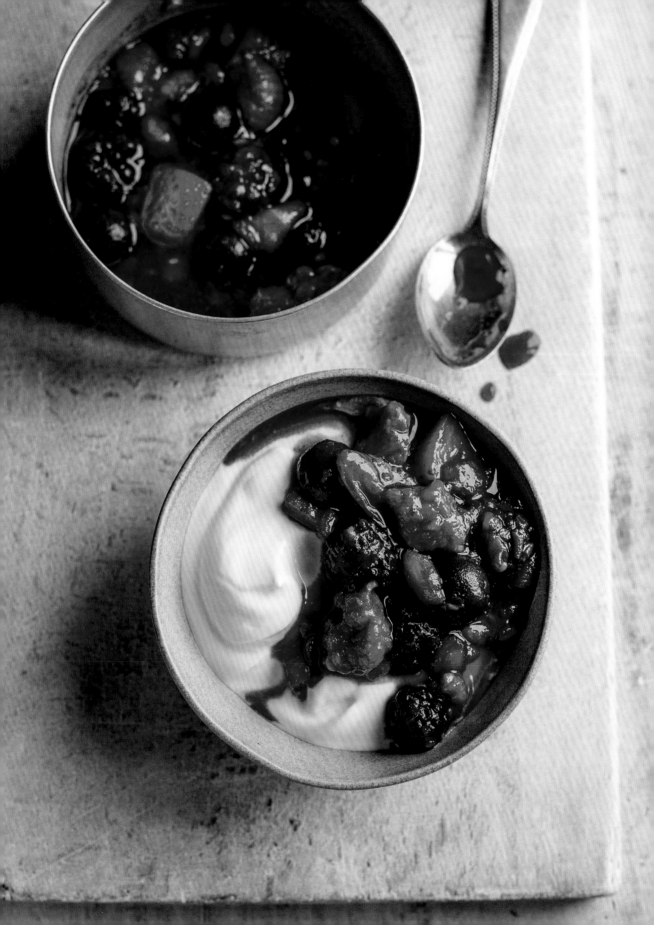

PER SERVING | **178cals** | PROTEIN **5.5g** | FAT **12.5g** | FIBRE **1g** | CARBS **10.5g**

Turmeric breakfast boost

SERVES 2

1 small banana, peeled
  and chopped (around
  65g prepared weight)
150g full-fat live Greek
  yoghurt
½–1 tsp ground turmeric
  (to taste)
¼ tsp ground ginger
¼ tsp ground cinnamon
8 pecan or walnut halves,
  roughly broken or chopped

NON-FAST DAYS
Serve with an extra sprinkling
of nuts.

This spiced, creamy yoghurt can be eaten for
breakfast or as a pudding. Either way you should
get the anti-inflammatory and cancer-reducing
benefits of turmeric, the effect of which is enhanced
by the fat in the yoghurt.

1 Place the banana in a bowl and mash roughly with a fork.

2 Add the yoghurt and sprinkle over the turmeric, ginger
and cinnamon.

3 Mix well, adding a splash of water if the yoghurt is a bit
thick, then divide between two dishes or glass tumblers,
sprinkle with the nuts and serve.

COOK'S TIP

★ Pecan nuts taste particularly delicious toasted. Simply
break into small pieces and dry fry in a small pan, without
any extra fat, for 2–3 minutes, or until lightly browned,
stirring constantly.

Banana and pecan muffin

SERVES 2

1 tbsp melted coconut oil
   or rapeseed oil
1 medium egg
1 small ripe banana,
   peeled and mashed
   with a fork (around
   65g prepared weight)
20g ground almonds
20g wholemeal
   self-raising flour
¼ tsp baking powder
8 pecan halves,
   roughly chopped
½ tsp ground cinnamon

You will need a microwave-proof mug (to hold around 350ml)

NON-FAST DAYS
Serve the muffin with a dollop of full-fat live Greek yoghurt.

A warm, fluffy breakfast treat that is a healthy alternative to a coffee-shop muffin. Serve with a handful of fresh berries, if you like (25g will add 11cals).

1 Use a tiny amount of the oil to lightly grease a microwave-proof mug.

2 Break the egg into the mug and beat really well with a fork.

3 Add the banana, ground almonds, flour, baking powder, pecans, cinnamon and the remaining oil and mix well.

4 Cook in a microwave on high for about 1½ minutes, or until risen and firm (the time will vary according to the wattage of your oven). The cake should have just begun to shrink back from the sides of the mug.

5 Leave to stand for 1 minute, then loosen the sides, tip the muffin out of the mug. Cut it in half and serve warm.

COOK'S TIPS

★ If you prefer to make two smaller muffins rather than one large one, you can combine the ingredients in a bowl and divide the mixture between two ramekin dishes.
★ You can melt the coconut oil in the microwave but don't let it overheat.

Minty citrus salad

SERVES 2

1 pink grapefruit
1 orange
1 clementine, tangerine
    or satsuma
4–5 fresh mint leaves,
    thinly sliced
100g full-fat live
    Greek yoghurt

NON-FAST DAYS
Scatter with 1 tablespoon
of toasted seeds.

This zingy, light and attractive breakfast could also be served as a dessert. You can prepare the fruit the night before and store in the fridge, so it's chilled and even more refreshing when you eat it.

1 Slice the ends off the grapefruit and orange and place them on a chopping board – ideally with a groove to catch any juice. Using a small sharp knife, cut off the peel and pith, working your way around both fruits. Turn the fruit on its side and slice thinly or separate into segments. Discard any pips.

2 Peel the clementine and thinly slice.

3 Divide the fruit between two plates and pour over any juices.

4 Scatter with the mint and serve with the Greek yoghurt.

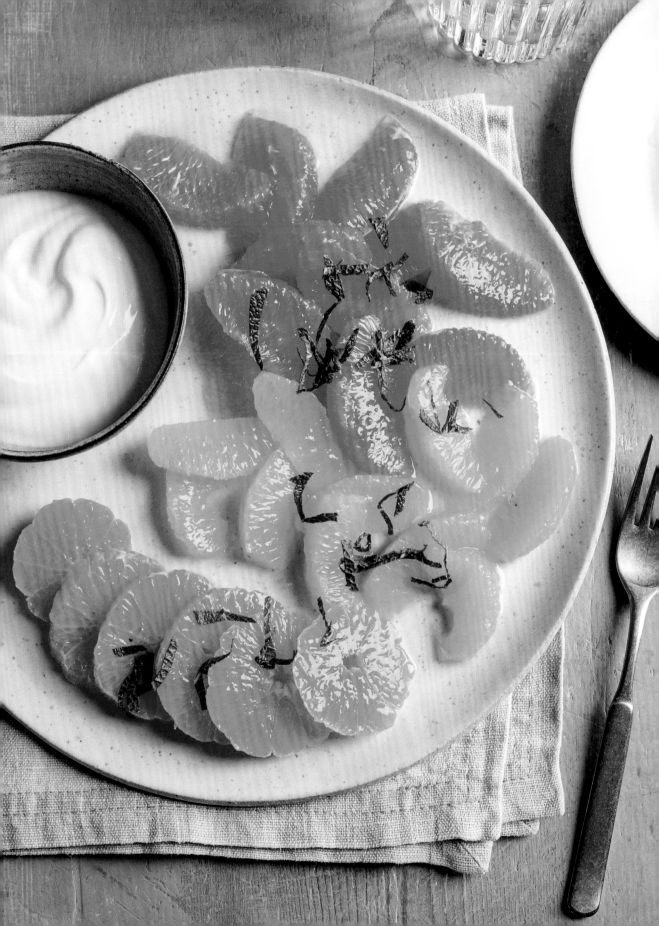

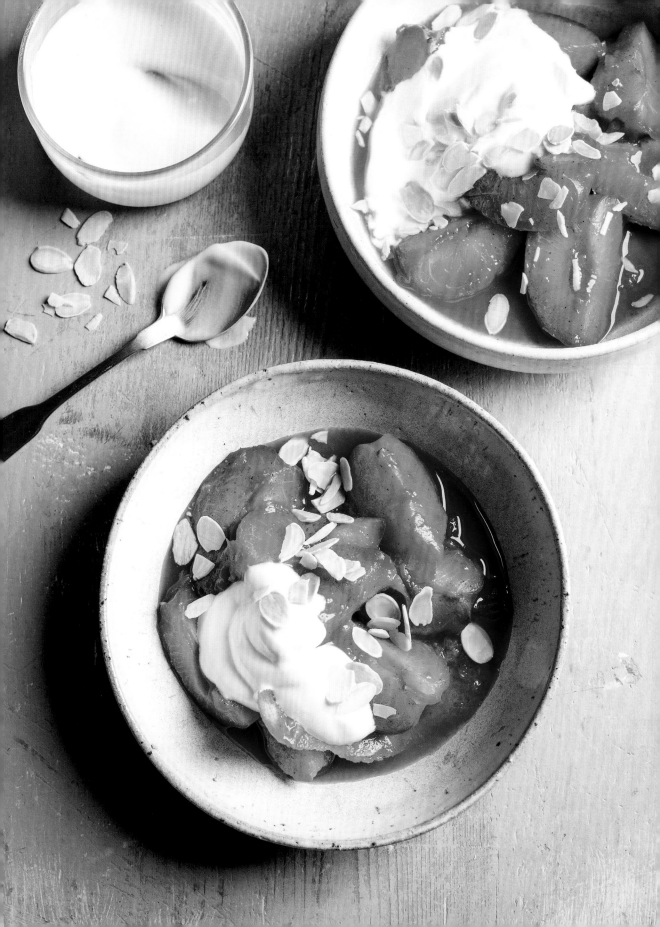

Spiced breakfast plums

SERVES 2

4 plums (around 275g),
halved and stoned
2 × 10–12cm strips orange
zest, removed with
a vegetable peeler
freshly squeezed juice
1 large orange
(around 100ml)
¼ tsp ground cinnamon
100g full-fat live
Greek yoghurt
15g toasted flaked almonds

NON-FAST DAYS
Add extra toasted nuts.

Delicious served warm or cold. This would also make a refreshing dessert.

1 Put the plums in a saucepan. Add the orange zest and juice, 150ml water and the cinnamon. Stir lightly.

2 Bring the liquid to a simmer, then cover with a lid, reduce the heat to low and cook for 10–15 minutes, or until the plums are soft but still holding their shape.

3 Divide the plums between two bowls and serve warm or cold with the Greek yoghurt and a sprinkling of toasted almonds.

COOK'S TIP

★ If you can't find ready-toasted almonds, toast your own (see page 18).

Poached eggs with mushrooms and spinach

SERVES 1

2 medium eggs, fridge cold
5g butter or 1 tsp olive oil
75g small chestnut
   mushrooms, sliced
large handful young
   spinach leaves

NON-FAST DAYS
Serve on top of a slice of
wholegrain buttered toast.

A quick, low-calorie but filling breakfast for
one. Make sure you use eggs that are very fresh.

1 Third fill a saucepan with water and bring to
a gentle simmer.

2 Break each egg into a cup, then carefully tip one
at a time into the pan. Cook over a very low heat, with
the water hardly bubbling, for about 3 minutes, or
until the whites are set but the yolks remain runny.

3 While the eggs are poaching, melt the butter or oil in
a non-stick frying pan over a medium heat and stir-fry the
mushrooms for 2–3 minutes or until lightly browned.

4 Add the spinach and toss with the mushrooms until
just wilted. Don't over-cook or lots of liquid will be
released. Season with a pinch of sea salt and a good
grinding of black pepper.

5 Spoon the mushrooms and spinach on to a warmed
plate. Drain the eggs with a slotted spoon and place on
top of the veg. Season with a little more ground black
pepper to serve.

COOK'S TIP

★ If you aren't using fridge-cold eggs, reduce the
cooking time slightly.

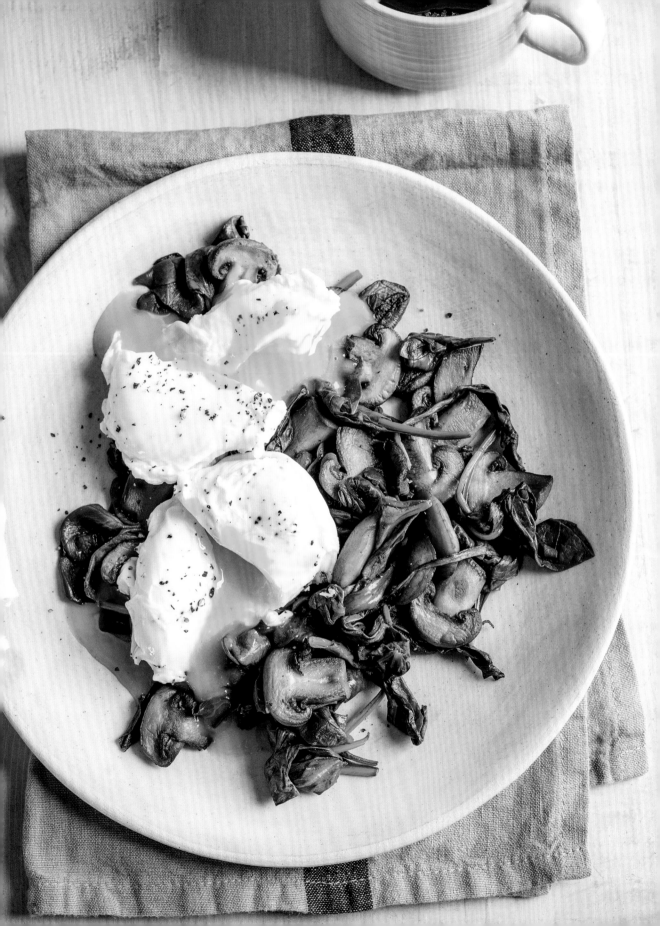

Smoked salmon omelette

SERVES 1

2 large eggs
1 tsp butter
1 tsp olive oil
50g smoked salmon slices,
    cut into thin strips
fresh chives, snipped,
    to serve (optional)

NON-FAST DAYS
Toss the salad with Simple salad dressing (see page 241) or a drizzle of extra-virgin olive oil and balsamic vinegar.

A luxurious, quick brunch (or lunch). The butter adds richness to the omelette, but you could just use the olive oil if you prefer. Serve with a mixed salad, adding the extra calories if dressed.

1 Break the eggs into a bowl and whisk thoroughly with a large whisk. Season with ground black pepper. (The salmon will be fairly salty, so there is no need to add salt.)

2 Melt the butter with the oil in a medium non-stick frying pan (approx. 19cm) over a medium heat. Pour the egg into the pan and let it cook for a few seconds. Using a wooden spoon, draw the egg in from the sides of the pan towards the centre and let the uncooked egg run to fill its place. Repeat this several times. This will make the omelette look thicker and lighter.

3 Sprinkle over the salmon strips and leave to cook for 1–2 minutes more, or until the omelette is lightly browned underneath and just set on top, and the salmon is warm and pale pink.

4 Slide the omelette on to a plate, fold and sprinkle with freshly snipped chives if using.

COOK'S TIPS

★ If you don't like smoked salmon, fry 100g sliced mushrooms in 1 tablespoon olive oil and use this instead. The mushroom version will contain 362cals per serving.
★ As an alternative you could lightly scramble the eggs instead and serve the salmon alongside.

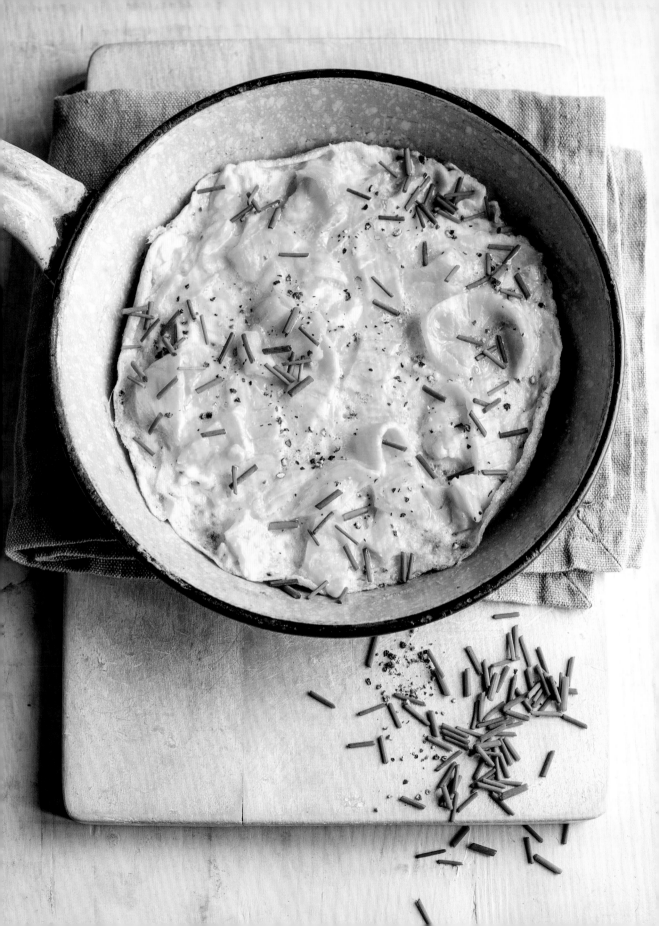

PER SERVING | **216cals** | PROTEIN **21g** | FAT **13g** | FIBRE **3g** | CARBS **2.5g**

Boiled eggs with long-stemmed soldiers

SERVES 1

2 large eggs, fridge cold
75g long-stemmed broccoli
  or asparagus, trimmed

NON-FAST DAYS
Serve with a slice of
seeded sourdough toast.

Lightly cooked long-stemmed broccoli or asparagus makes a fab alternative to toast soldiers.

1 Half fill a small saucepan with water and bring to the boil. Using a slotted spoon, gently add the eggs to the water one at a time and cook for 6–7 minutes for a soft-boiled egg.

2 Meanwhile, fill a wide-based pan with water until around 5cm deep and bring to a simmer. Cook the broccoli or asparagus for 4–5 minutes, or until just tender. Drain.

3 Place the eggs in egg cups on a small plate and serve with the warm stems for dipping.

COOK'S TIP

★ If you aren't using fridge-cold eggs, reduce the cooking time by around 1 minute.

Mushrooms on toasted sourdough

SERVES 1

1 tbsp olive oil
140g Portobello mushrooms
   (around 2 large), sliced
1 thin slice wholegrain
   sourdough bread
   (around 20g)
½ garlic clove, peeled
   and crushed
2 tsp fresh thyme leaves
   or ¼ tsp dried thyme
1 tsp balsamic vinegar
small handful fresh parsley,
   leaves roughly chopped
2 thin slices goat's cheese
   (around 40g)

NON-FAST DAYS
Serve with extra slices of goat's cheese and a drizzle of olive oil.

A simple and very quick meal, full of flavour and easy to multiply for extra servings. It takes almost as little time to cook the mushrooms as it does to toast the bread.

1 Heat the oil in large non-stick frying pan over a high heat and fry the mushrooms for 3 minutes, or until lightly browned, stirring constantly.

2 Meanwhile, toast the bread.

3 Add the garlic and thyme to the mushrooms and cook for 30 seconds, stirring. Add the vinegar and parsley and toss together briefly.

4 Pile the mushrooms on to the toast, top with the goat's cheese and finish with a generous grind of black pepper.

COOK'S TIP

★ We recommend keeping bread ready-sliced in the freezer because, if it is put away, it encourages you to cut down on it and just eat it as an occasional treat. You also get the benefit of reducing the starchy calories in the bread – freezing converts some of the starchy carbohydrates (which are not so good) into resistant starch, which *is* good as it is less digestible (see page 243 for more on this). If you can't get hold of sourdough bread, any wholegrain will do, or any bread made with traditional grains, such as spelt or rye.

Smashed avocado on toast

SERVES 2

2 thin slices wholegrain
   sourdough bread
   (each around 20g)
1 ripe medium avocado,
   stoned, peeled and roughly
   chopped (about 75g prepared
   weight – see tip below)
25g walnut halves (around 10),
   roughly chopped
1 plump red chilli, deseeded
   and diced, or a pinch of
   crushed dried chilli flakes
   (optional)
2 tsp balsamic vinegar

NON-FAST DAYS
Top the avocado toast with
one or two freshly poached
eggs, or some crumbled feta.
A tablespoon of toasted mixed
seeds is also a lovely addition.

This super-fast breakfast is a great way of using
up avocados that are over-ripe.

1 Toast the bread and divide between two plates
(or serve on one plate to share).

2 Place the avocado and walnuts in a small bowl and
mash with a fork.

3 Spread on to the hot toast, sprinkle with the chilli,
if using, and drizzle with the balsamic vinegar. Season
with sea salt and ground black pepper to serve.

COOK'S TIPS

★ We've found the best way to prepare an avocado is to cut
it in half, remove the stone, and then, using a large serving
spoon, scoop between the skin and the flesh and lift the half
avocado out in one piece. Turn it on its cut side and slice
or chop, as needed.
★ If you can't get hold of sourdough bread, any wholegrain
will do.

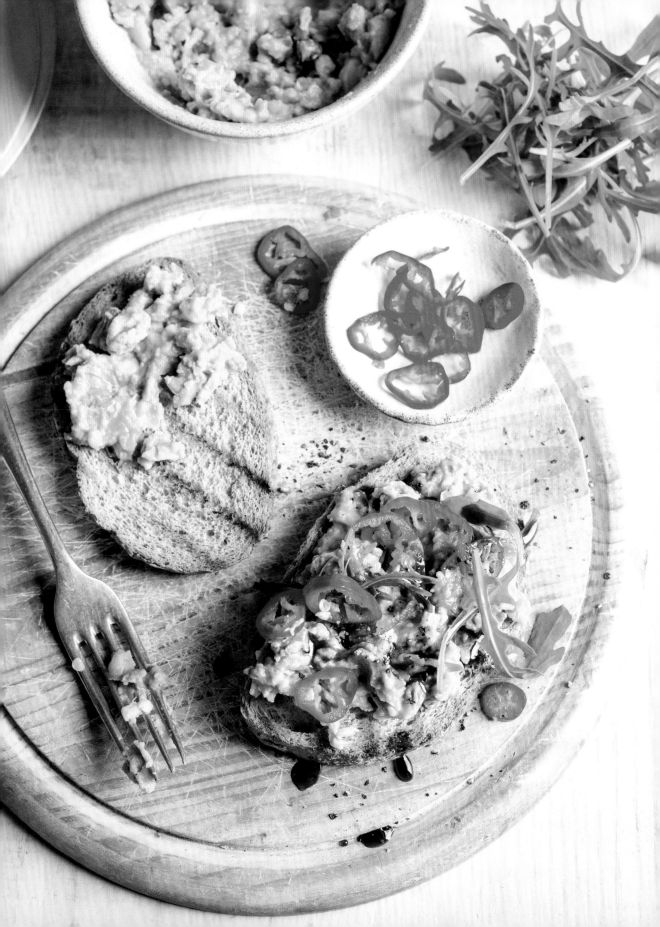

PER SERVING | **312cals** | PROTEIN **19.5g** | FAT **17g** | FIBRE **5.5g** | CARBS **17.5g**

Shakshuka

SERVES 2

1 tbsp olive oil

1 medium red onion, peeled and finely chopped

1 yellow pepper, deseeded and thinly sliced

2 garlic cloves, peeled and crushed

1 tsp ground cumin

½–1 tsp hot smoked paprika (to taste)

1 × 400g can chopped tomatoes

1 tbsp tomato purée

4 medium eggs

small handful fresh coriander or flat-leaf parsley, leaves roughly chopped, to serve (optional)

NON-FAST DAYS
Crumble feta over the top after adding the eggs and serve with warmed wholemeal pitta bread.

A hugely popular brunch dish from the Middle East and North Africa made with eggs poached in a lightly spiced tomato sauce.

1 Heat the oil in a medium non-stick frying pan or shallow casserole that has a lid, add the onion and pepper and gently fry for 5–6 minutes, or until softened, stirring regularly.

2 Add the garlic, cumin and paprika and cook for 20–30 seconds, stirring.

3 Tip the tomatoes into the pan, add the tomato purée, a good pinch of sea salt and lots of ground black pepper.

4 Bring to a simmer and cook for about 4 minutes, or until the tomato sauce has thickened, stirring regularly.

5 Make four holes in the vegetable mixture and break an egg into each one. Cover the pan with the lid and cook very gently for 3–5 minutes, or until the whites are set but the yolks remain runny.

6 Sprinkle with the fresh herbs, if using, and season with more ground black pepper to serve.

COOK'S TIP

★ If your frying pan doesn't have a lid, use a large heatproof plate (take care when you remove it as it will be extremely hot) or use a large piece of kitchen foil. Covering the pan helps the eggs cook and prevents the tomato sauce from becoming too thick.

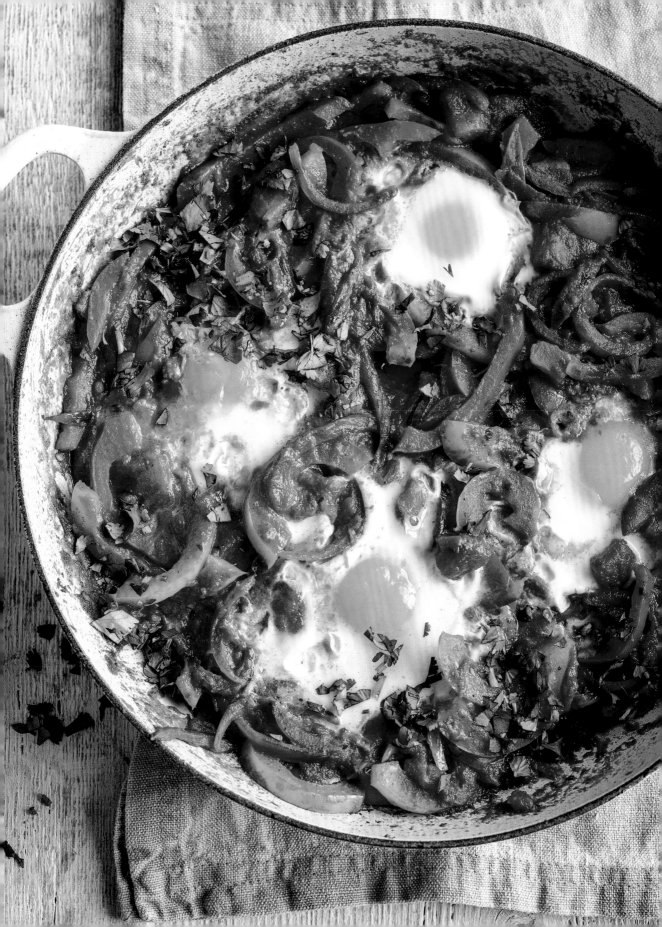

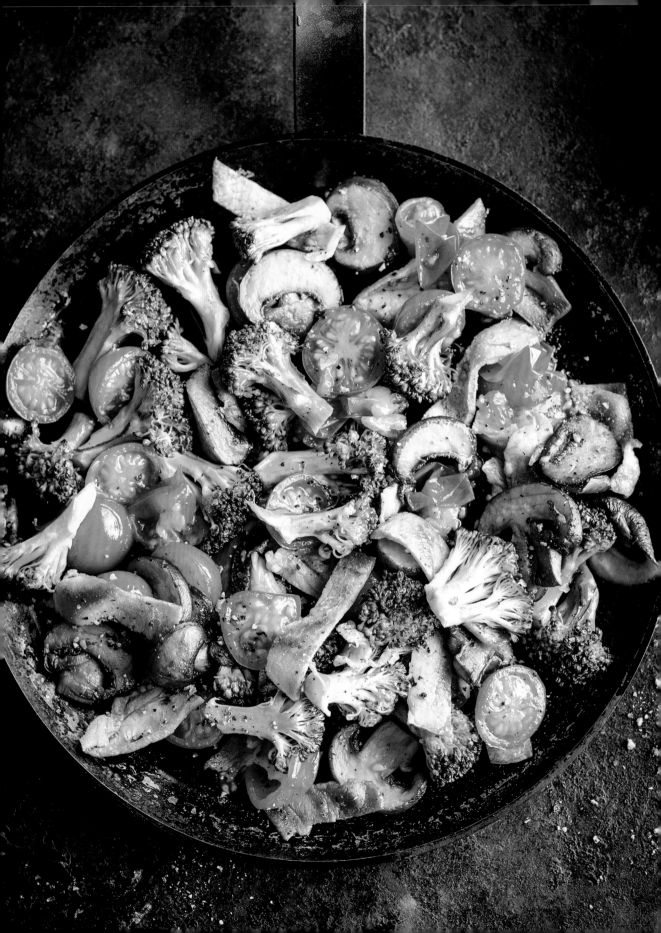

Bacon, broccoli, tomato and mushroom fry-up

SERVES 2

100g broccoli, cut into
    small florets
1 tbsp olive or rapeseed oil
2 rashers smoked back bacon,
    trimmed of the fat then
    cut into wide strips
100g chestnut mushrooms,
    sliced
10 cherry tomatoes, halved

NON-FAST DAYS
Push the broccoli and bacon
mixture to one side of the pan,
add a little more oil and fry
a couple of eggs.

A handy breakfast or brunch that takes less than
10 minutes to prepare. Although processed meats,
such as bacon, should be eaten in moderation,
this makes a delicious weekend treat.

1 Third fill a saucepan with water and bring to the boil.
Add the broccoli and return to the boil. Cook for 3 minutes,
then drain.

2 Meanwhile, heat the oil in a large non-stick frying pan
and fry the bacon, mushrooms and tomatoes for 2 minutes,
or until the mushrooms are lightly browned.

3 Add the broccoli and cook for 1 minute more, stirring.

4 Divide between two plates, season with ground black
pepper and serve.

Cowboy baked beans

SERVES 2

1 tbsp olive oil

1 small onion, peeled and
    very finely chopped

1 garlic clove, peeled
    and crushed

1 tsp smoked paprika,
    hot or sweet,
    depending on taste

1 × 400g can haricot
    beans, drained

350g passata

1 tbsp Worcestershire sauce

2 thin slices wholegrain
    bread (each around 20g)

NON-FAST DAYS
Serve with an extra slice
of wholegrain toast and
a generous drizzle of
olive oil.

Homemade baked beans are a favourite of ours.
This simple version can be served at breakfast or
as an accompaniment to grilled chicken or meat.
It's also lovely topped with crumbled cheese for
a quick supper.

1 Heat the oil in a non-stick saucepan, add the onion
and gently fry for 3–4 minutes, or until soft.

2 Add the garlic and paprika and cook for a few seconds
more, stirring.

3 Tip the beans into the pan and add the passata and
Worcestershire sauce. Season with sea salt and ground
black pepper. Bring to a gentle simmer and cook for
5 minutes, or until the sauce is thickened, stirring
regularly, especially towards the end of the cooking time.

4 Just before the beans are ready, toast the bread and
place on two plates. Spoon the beans over and serve.

COOK'S TIP

★ Use any canned beans you like; just keep the quantities
the same.

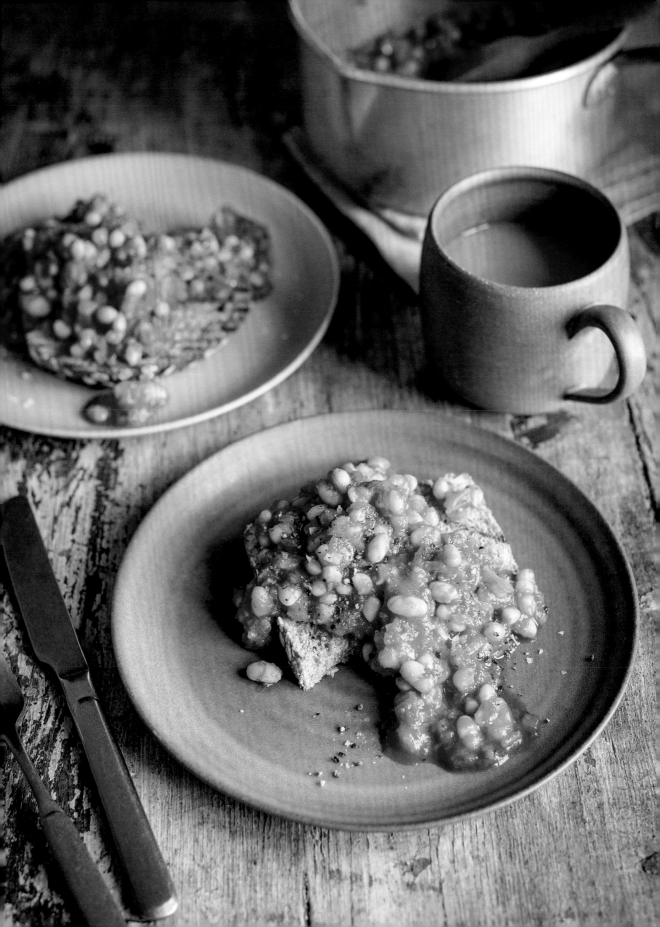

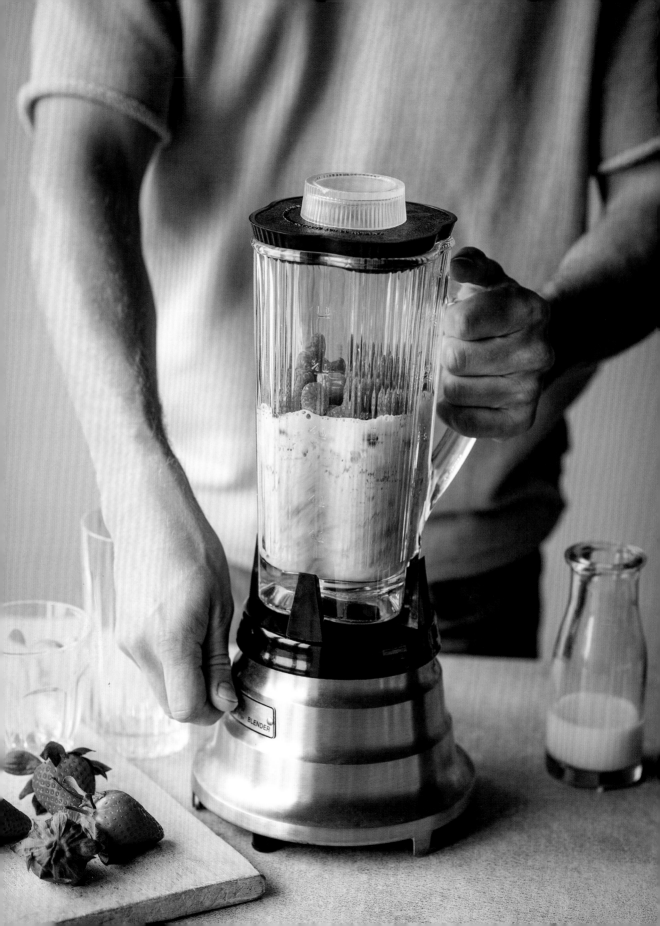

Shakes
and Soups

Although we recommend real food first, we know that shakes can be very useful as meal replacements to help keep you on track. Do try one of our delicious recipes here. They are likely to be healthier than those you buy in shops and online, which tend to be high in sugar and starchy carbs. NB If you are not using dairy, we suggest adding unsweetened almond milk (13cals per 100ml) or oat milk (44cals per 100ml).

Our soups, meanwhile, are as tasty as they are filling. The recipes mainly serve four so you can take one portion to work for lunch and store extra portions in the fridge for a few days or put them in the freezer. Make soups your fast-day friend.

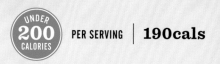
Shakes

Making these shakes is easy.

SERVES 1

1 Put all the ingredients in a blender and blitz until smooth. Add more water, if necessary, to reach your preferred consistency.

2 Pour into a glass to serve.

Iced berry shake

Choose any frozen fruit you like for this cool shake. Make sure your blender is sturdy enough to crush ice.

25g full-fat live Greek yoghurt
75ml semi-skimmed milk
40g frozen mixed berries,
   such as strawberries and blueberries
½ medium banana (around 50g peeled weight),
   peeled and roughly chopped
1 tbsp jumbo porridge oats
5g ground almonds
2 tbsp cold water

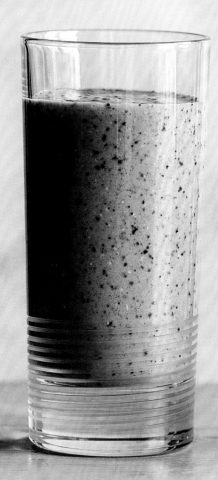

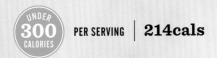

UNDER 300 CALORIES | PER SERVING | **214cals**

UNDER 200 CALORIES | PER SERVING | **195cals**

Nutty banana shake

Use no-added-sugar nut butter for this creamy-tasting shake.

20g full-fat live Greek yoghurt
100ml semi-skimmed milk
½ medium banana (around
    50g peeled weight), peeled
    and roughly chopped
15g no-added-sugar cashew
    or almond nut butter
2 tbsp cold water

Chocolate and strawberry shake

A delicious and filling chocolaty hit.

100ml semi-skimmed milk
25g full-fat live Greek yoghurt
100g fresh or frozen strawberries
15g jumbo porridge oats
1 soft pitted date
1 tsp cocoa powder
2 tbsp cold water

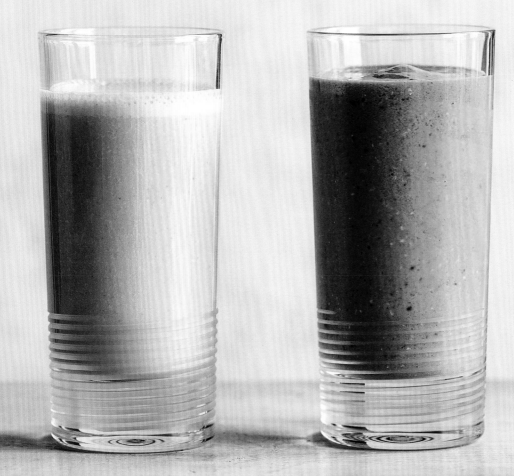

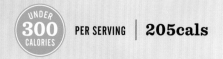
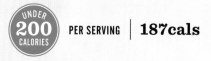

Minted avocado and cucumber shake

A creamy shake with a refreshing hint of mint.

½ medium avocado, stoned, peeled and quartered (about 75g prepared weight – see tip on page 40)
200g cucumber, thickly sliced
25g young spinach leaves
12 fresh mint leaves
15g full-fat live Greek yoghurt
100ml cold water

Orange, carrot and cashew shake

This makes a zingy drink with a vibrant orange colour. Make sure your blender is sturdy enough to cope with the carrot slices.

2 medium carrots (around 170g), trimmed and sliced
½ medium orange, peeled and cut into chunky pieces
15g no-added-sugar cashew nut butter or almond butter
125ml cold water

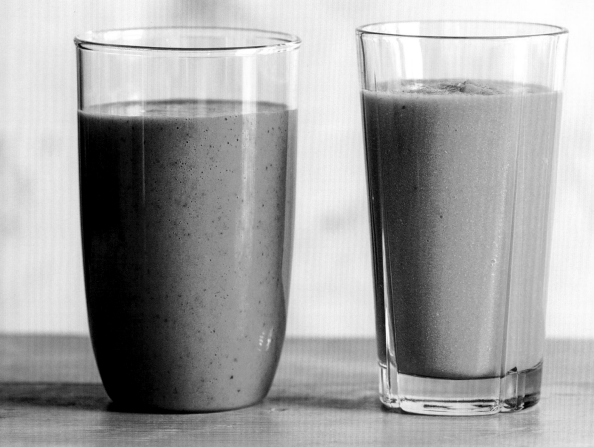

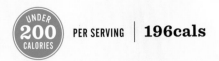

Green ginger shake

Crisp green apple adds fibre and sweetness to this gorgeous green shake. Use a red-skinned apple if you prefer.

1 green apple, quartered and cored
½ medium courgette (around 65g), trimmed and thickly sliced
8g fresh root ginger, peeled and roughly chopped
½ tsp ground turmeric
10g mixed seeds (such as sunflower, pumpkin, sesame and flax)
2 tsp extra-virgin olive oil
100ml cold water

Gazpacho-style shake

This is lovely served cold with a couple of ice cubes.

100g cucumber, roughly chopped
2–3 ripe vine tomatoes (around 125g), quartered
½ red pepper, deseeded and sliced
¼ small red onion (around 20g), peeled
25g full-fat live Greek yoghurt
10g ground almonds
1 tbsp tomato purée
1 tsp extra-virgin olive oil
2 tbsp cold water
sea salt and freshly ground black pepper, to taste

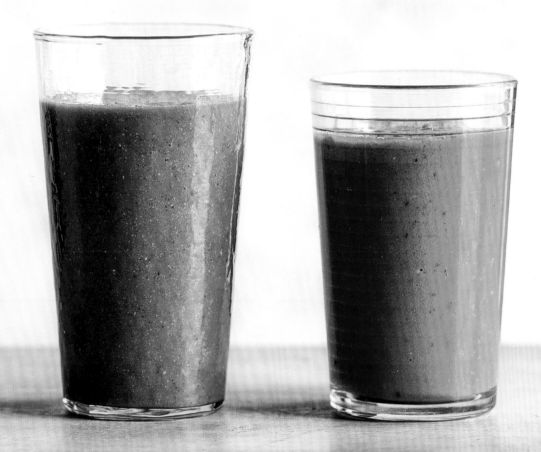

PER SERVING | **249cals** | PROTEIN **7g** | FAT **14.5g** | FIBRE **8g** | CARBS **18.5g**

Bean soup with kale and pesto

SERVES 4

2 tbsp olive oil

1 medium onion, peeled
    and roughly chopped

1 celery stick, cut into
    roughly 1cm chunks

2 medium carrots,
    trimmed and cut into
    roughly 1cm chunks

1 medium courgette, trimmed,
    halved lengthways and cut
    into roughly 1cm slices

1 × 400g can cannellini beans,
    drained

1 × 400g can borlotti
    or kidney beans, drained

1 vegetable or chicken
    stock cube

75g kale or dark green cabbage,
    thickly sliced and tough
    stalks discarded

60g fresh basil pesto

NON-FAST DAYS

Serve with a drizzle of olive
oil and toasted wholegrain
or sourdough bread. For extra
sustenance, add some diced
fried halloumi or bacon.

Super-quick and easy, this tastes fabulous topped
with the fresh basil pesto. You can use any of your
favourite beans – just keep the quantities the same.

1 Heat the oil in a large non-stick saucepan, add the onion,
celery, carrots and courgette and gently fry for 10 minutes,
stirring occasionally.

2 Tip the beans into the pan, add the stock cube and
1.2 litres water and stir to dissolve. Add the kale or cabbage
and bring to a simmer. Cook for 5–7 minutes, stirring
occasionally, until the vegetables are tender.

3 Season with sea salt and ground black pepper to taste,
then ladle into warmed bowls and top with the pesto.

COOK'S TIP

★ You'll find tubs of fresh basil pesto in the chilled
department of the supermarket, usually with the fresh
pasta, but you can use the jarred kind as well.

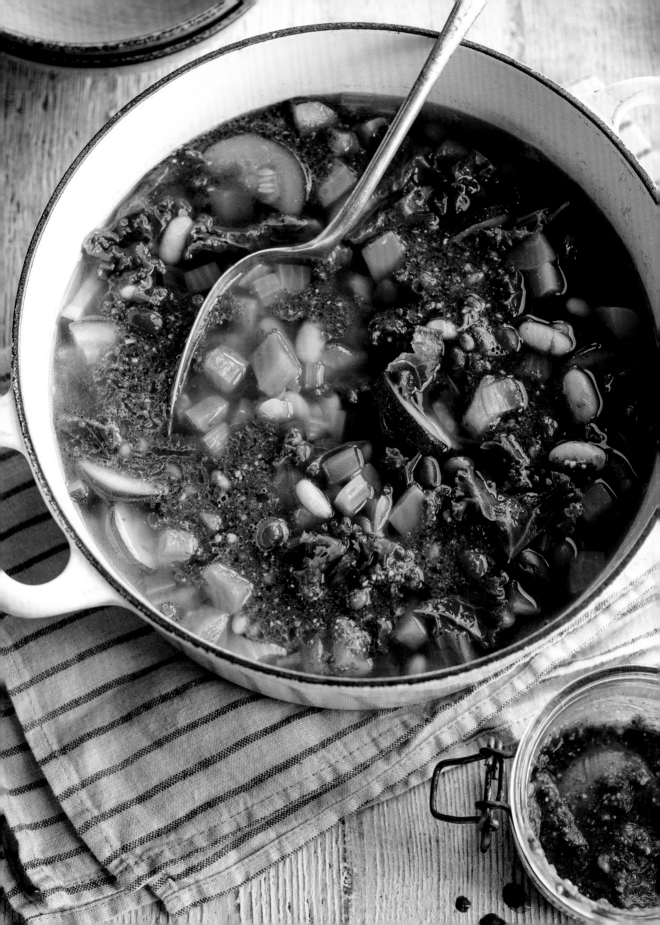

Broccoli and blue cheese soup

SERVES 4

1 tbsp olive or rapeseed oil

1 medium onion, peeled and finely chopped

1 large head broccoli (around 400g), roughly chopped, including the stalk

1 vegetable or chicken stock cube

75g soft blue cheese, such as Roquefort

NON-FAST DAYS

Fry 4 rashers smoked streaky bacon in a dry pan until crisp. Break into small pieces and sprinkle on to the soup just before serving with a slice of toasted wholegrain bread.

A rich, comforting soup that is good for the bugs in your gut, too.

1 Heat the oil in a large non-stick saucepan, add the onion and gently fry for 5 minutes, or until softened, stirring regularly.

2 Add the broccoli and crumble the stock cube over the top. Pour in 1 litre water and bring to the boil. Reduce the heat and simmer for 10 minutes, or until the broccoli is very tender, stirring occasionally.

3 Remove from the heat and blitz with a stick blender or cool slightly and blend in a food processor until smooth.

4 Return to the heat, stir in most of the cheese and adjust the seasoning to taste. Warm through gently, adding a little extra water if needed, before serving with the remaining cheese crumbled on top.

COOK'S TIP

★ If you have odds and ends of cauliflower, use these up with the broccoli – just keep to around 400g total weight.

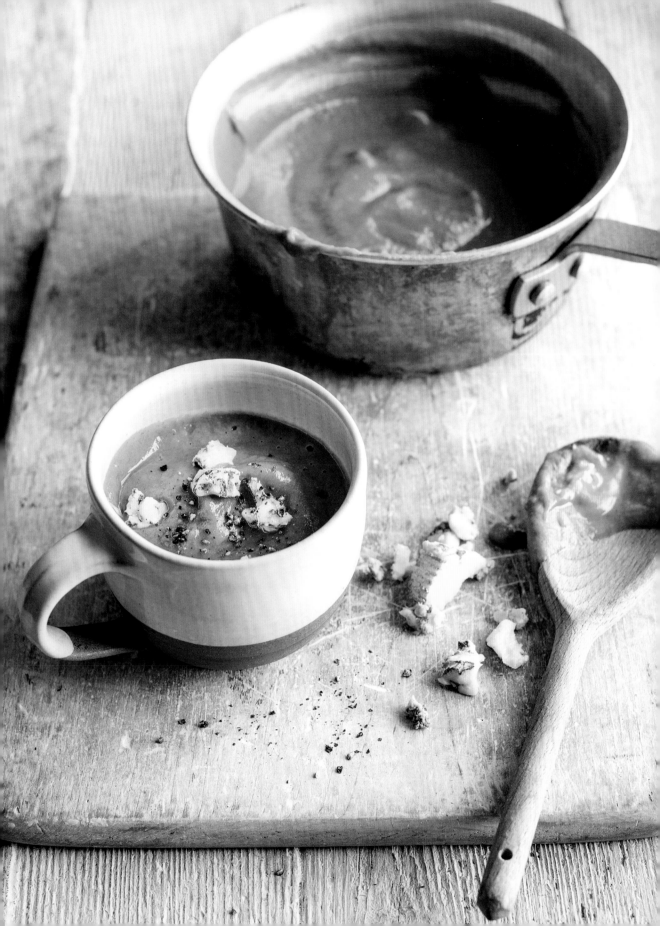

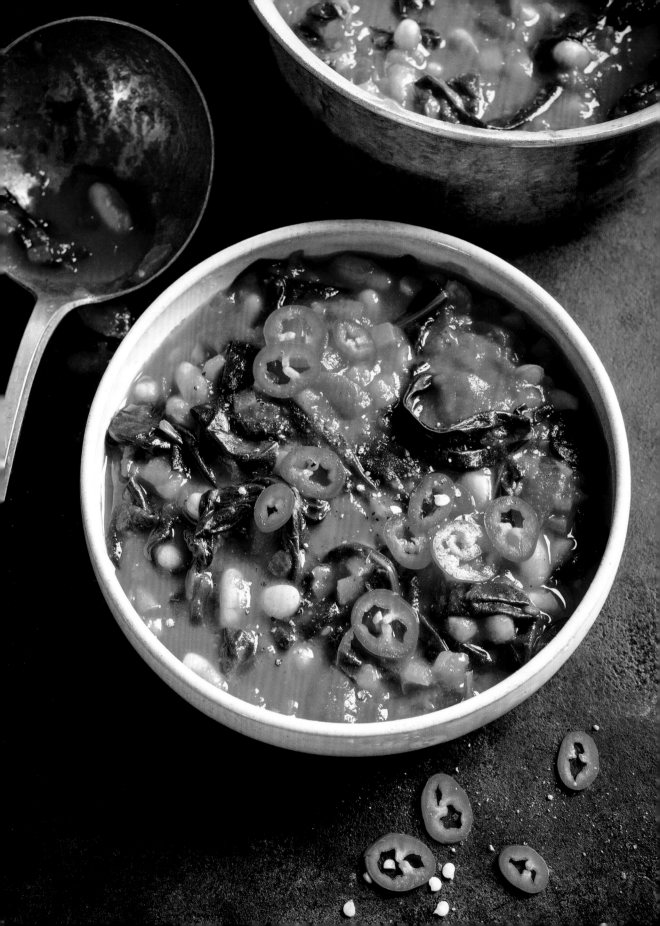

Spiced bean and spinach soup

SERVES 3

1 tbsp olive oil
1 medium onion, peeled
　and finely chopped
1 large garlic clove,
　peeled and crushed
1 tsp ground cumin
1 tbsp harissa paste
1 × 400g can chopped tomatoes
1 × 400g can cannellini beans,
　drained and rinsed
1 vegetable stock cube
200g frozen spinach

NON-FAST DAYS
Scatter some diced cooked
bacon into the soup for added
protein, along with a good glug
of olive oil. Serve it with a
chunk of wholegrain bread.

Made from ingredients you can keep in your
cupboards and freezer, this is a soup to power
you through the day. Harissa is a spiced red pepper
and chilli paste that you should find in the World
Foods section of the supermarket.

1 Heat the oil in a large non-stick saucepan, add the
onion and gently fry for 5 minutes, or until softened,
stirring regularly.

2 Add the garlic, cumin and harissa paste and cook
for a few seconds more, stirring.

3 Tip the tomatoes and cannellini beans into the pan
and crumble over the stock cube. Add 500ml water and
stir in the frozen spinach. Bring the liquid to a simmer
(this may take a while as the spinach will need to thaw),
then leave to cook for 10 minutes, stirring regularly,
adding a little extra water if needed.

4 Season with sea salt and ground black pepper to serve.

COOK'S TIP

★ Add a finely sliced fresh chilli or ½ teaspoon crushed
dried chilli flakes before serving for an extra kick.
A tablespoon of tomato purée stirred in at the same time
as the tomatoes will bring extra richness to the soup
for just an additional 5cals per serving.

PER SERVING | **192cals** | PROTEIN **8g** | FAT **7.5g** | FIBRE **6.5g** | CARBS **20g**

Speedy tomato soup

SERVES 2

1 × 400g can chopped tomatoes
½ × 400g can cannellini
    beans, drained
2 spring onions, trimmed
    and roughly chopped
30g full-fat live Greek yoghurt
6 large basil leaves, plus
    extra to serve (optional)
1 tbsp olive oil
1 tbsp tomato purée

An instant lunch or supper, with beans to make
it more filling.

1 Place all the ingredients in a blender, season with sea
salt and lots of ground black pepper and blitz until smooth.

2 Transfer to a non-stick saucepan, stir in enough water to
reach your preferred consistency and heat through gently.

3 Season to taste and pour into bowls or mugs to serve
with basil leaves to garnish, if you like.

NON-FAST DAYS
Serve with a slice of wholegrain
or seeded sourdough bread.
Add a tablespoon of cooked diced
bacon or chorizo to the soup for
added flavour and protein, and
a liberal drizzle of olive oil.

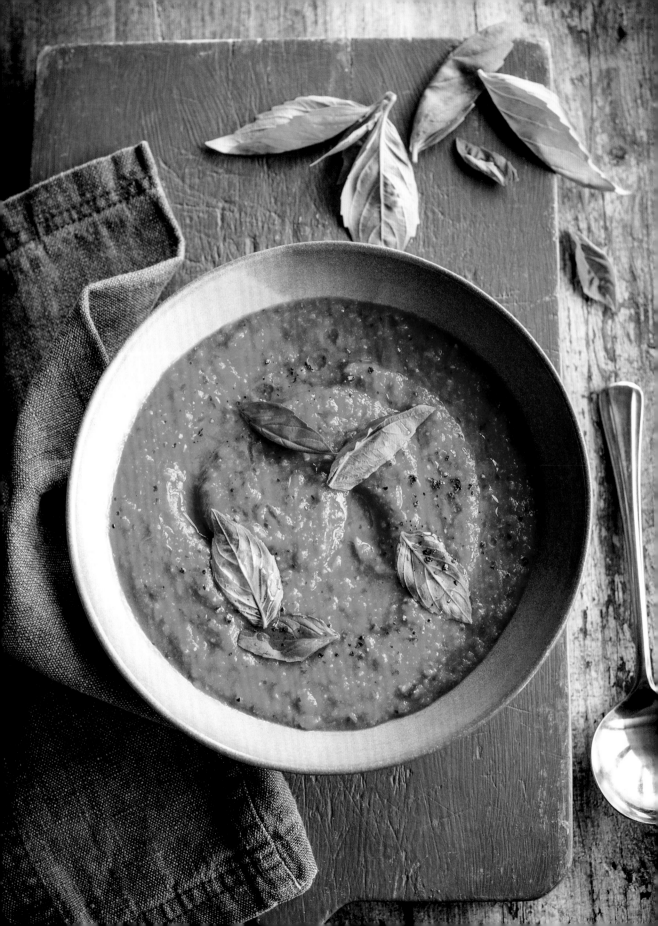

Almost instant noodle soup

SERVES 2

50g dried wholewheat noodles
   or soba buckwheat noodles
4 tsp miso paste
20g fresh root ginger,
   peeled and finely grated
2 tbsp dark soy sauce
4–6 chestnut mushrooms,
   depending on size (around
   75g), very finely sliced
large handful young
   spinach leaves
4 spring onions, trimmed
   and very finely sliced
½ tsp crushed dried
   chilli flakes
25g roasted cashew nuts,
   roughly chopped
2 large handfuls fresh
   coriander, leaves
   roughly chopped

NON-FAST DAYS
Add extra protein, such
as shredded cooked chicken
or cubes of tofu.

A delicious, Asian-inspired soup, which works
particularly well as a lunch on the go.

1 Half fill a saucepan with water and bring to the boil. Add
the noodles, return to the boil and cook for 3–4 minutes
until tender, or according to the pack instructions. Pour
the noodles into a sieve and rinse under cold running
water. Drain well.

2 Divide the miso paste, ginger and soy sauce between two
large heatproof jars (or other heatproof lidded containers).

3 Place the mushrooms on top, then add – in the following
order – the cooked noodles, spinach, spring onions, chilli
flakes, cashews and coriander. Cover and keep chilled.

4 When ready to serve, add 250–300ml just-boiled water
from a kettle (roughly a mug full) to each jar. The water
should rise about halfway up the ingredients. Cover loosely
and leave to stand for 2 minutes to allow the vegetables
to soften and the noodles to heat.

5 Stir well, leave to stand for a further 1–2 minutes then
serve immediately.

COOK'S TIPS

★ The just-boiled water will warm the ingredients but
they won't be hot, so you could give the soup a quick blast
in a microwave to heat it further. Make sure your container
is suitable for microwave cooking. You could also heat the
soup in a pan.
★ Dry noodles come in different-sized bundles – do your
best to keep as close to 50g as possible.

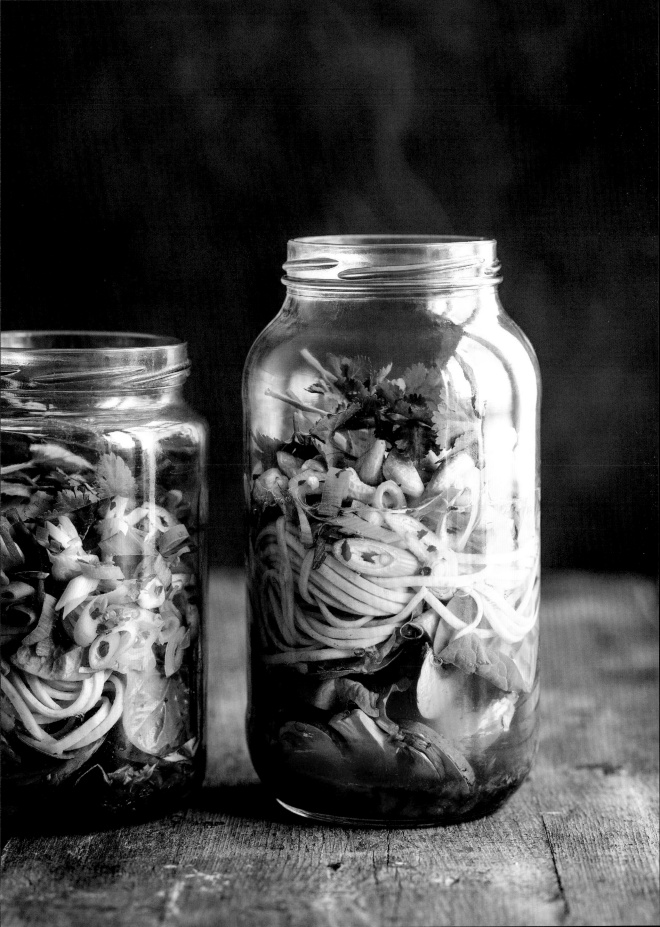

Creamy mushroom soup

SERVES 4

1 tbsp olive oil

1 large onion, peeled and
    roughly chopped

300g chestnut mushrooms
    or Portobello mushrooms,
    sliced

2 large garlic cloves,
    peeled and crushed

1 vegetable or chicken
    stock cube

75ml full-fat milk

NON-FAST DAYS

Serve with a slice of toasted
wholegrain or sourdough
bread and drizzle generously
with olive oil.

A luxurious, creamy mushroom soup that's incredibly
easy to make and marvellously low in calories. Don't
skip any of the cooking stages: they all help add flavour.

1 Heat the oil in a large non-stick saucepan, add the onion
and gently fry for 5 minutes, or until softened and lightly
browned, stirring regularly.

2 Add the mushrooms and garlic and cook for 5 minutes,
stirring regularly. (Don't allow the garlic to burn or it
will taste bitter.)

3 Crumble in the stock cube and pour in 600ml water.
Season with sea salt and lots of ground black pepper. Bring
to the boil, then reduce the heat and simmer for 10 minutes,
stirring occasionally.

4 Remove from the heat and blitz with a stick blender or
cool slightly and blend in a food processor until smooth.

5 Stir in the milk, return to the heat and adjust the seasoning
to taste. Add a little extra milk or water to reach your
preferred consistency and warm through before serving.

COOK'S TIP

★ Swap the milk for a dairy-free alternative if you like.
There are 47cals in 75ml full-fat milk so remember to
adjust the total calories.

Clear chicken and pea soup

SERVES 2

1 tbsp olive oil
1 small onion, peeled
   and finely chopped
150g leftover cooked chicken,
   roughly chopped
500ml fresh chicken stock
   (see below)
150g frozen peas

NON-FAST DAYS
Serve with warmed wholegrain
bread and top with spoonfuls of
sun-dried tomato or basil pesto.

This simple soup makes great use of the leftovers from
a roast chicken or turkey. If you don't have fresh stock,
use a good-quality chicken stock cube instead. Stir in
chopped fresh parsley or tarragon leaves if you like.

1 Heat the oil in a non-stick saucepan, add the onion and
gently fry for 3–4 minutes, or until softened, stirring regularly.

2 Add the chicken, stock and peas, season with ground
black pepper and bring to a simmer. Cook for 5 minutes,
stirring occasionally.

3 Divide between two warmed bowls and serve.

COOK'S TIP

★ To make the chicken stock, put the carcass from a roasted
chicken in a large saucepan after removing the skin. Add
a quartered onion, 2 thickly sliced carrots, 2 thickly sliced
sticks of celery, 1 bay leaf and ¼ teaspoon dried thyme
(or a small bunch of fresh thyme). Add 1 teaspoon sea salt
and 10 peppercorns. Bring the liquid to a very gentle
simmer – do not allow to boil – cover the pan with a lid
and cook for 1–4 hours, to release the nutrients. Drain
first through a colander and then a sieve. Let it cool, then
cover and keep in the fridge for up to 2 days, if not using
immediately, or freeze for up to 3 months.

PER SERVING | **223cals** | PROTEIN **20.5g** | FAT **8g** | FIBRE **4.5g** | CARBS **15.5g**

Curried chicken and lentil soup

SERVES 4

1 tbsp olive or coconut oil
1 medium onion, peeled and
    finely chopped
1 pepper, any colour,
    deseeded and cut into
    roughly 1.5cm chunks
2 tbsp medium curry powder
1 × 400g can chopped tomatoes
1 chicken stock cube
50g dried red split lentils
225g frozen spinach
200g cooked chicken,
    roughly chopped
lemon wedges, to serve

NON-FAST DAYS
Top with a couple of tablespoons
of toasted almonds and serve
with a spoonful of full-fat live
Greek yoghurt or Minty yoghurt
raitha (see page 106).

Lentils and spinach add plenty of fibre to this soup,
making it particularly filling.

1 Heat the oil in a large non-stick saucepan, add the onion
and pepper and gently fry for 5 minutes, or until softened.
Stir in the curry powder and cook for a few seconds more.

2 Add the tomatoes and bring to the boil. Keep stirring for
a couple of minutes, then crumble over the chicken stock
cube and add 1 litre water.

3 Rinse the lentils and add to the pan, along with the frozen
spinach, and bring to a simmer. Season well with sea salt
and lots of ground black pepper. Cook for 10 minutes,
stirring regularly.

4 Add the chicken pieces and cook for 8–10 minutes more,
or until the lentils are soft and the spinach is completely
thawed, stirring regularly. Add extra water if the soup
thickens too much.

5 Adjust the seasoning to taste and serve in deep bowls
with lemon wedges for squeezing over.

COOK'S TIP

★ To make a vegetarian version: use a vegetable stock
cube and replace the chicken with Quorn pieces. The
chicken contains 178cals per 100g, so you'll need to
adjust the calories accordingly.

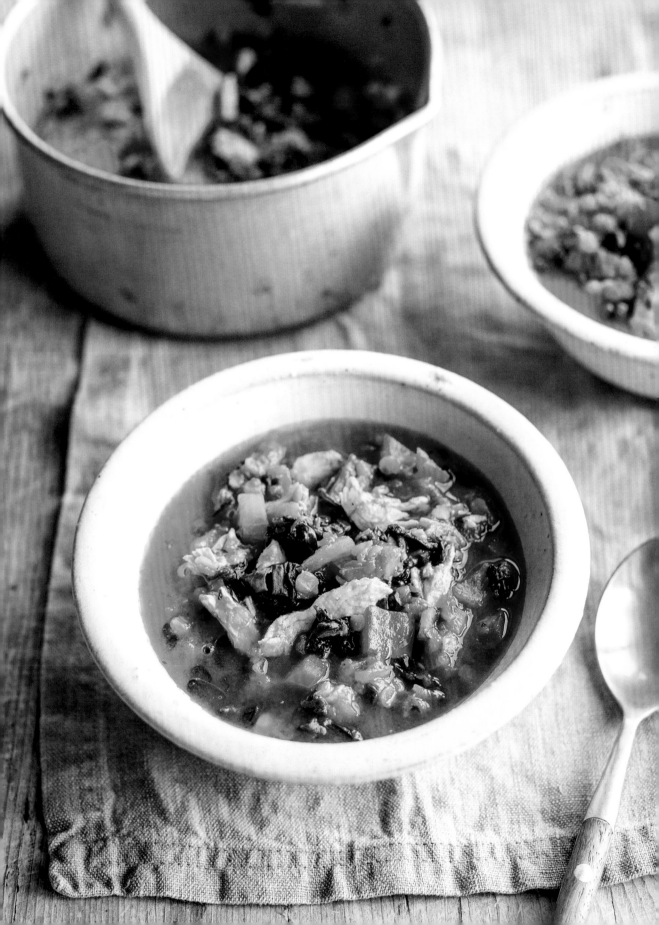

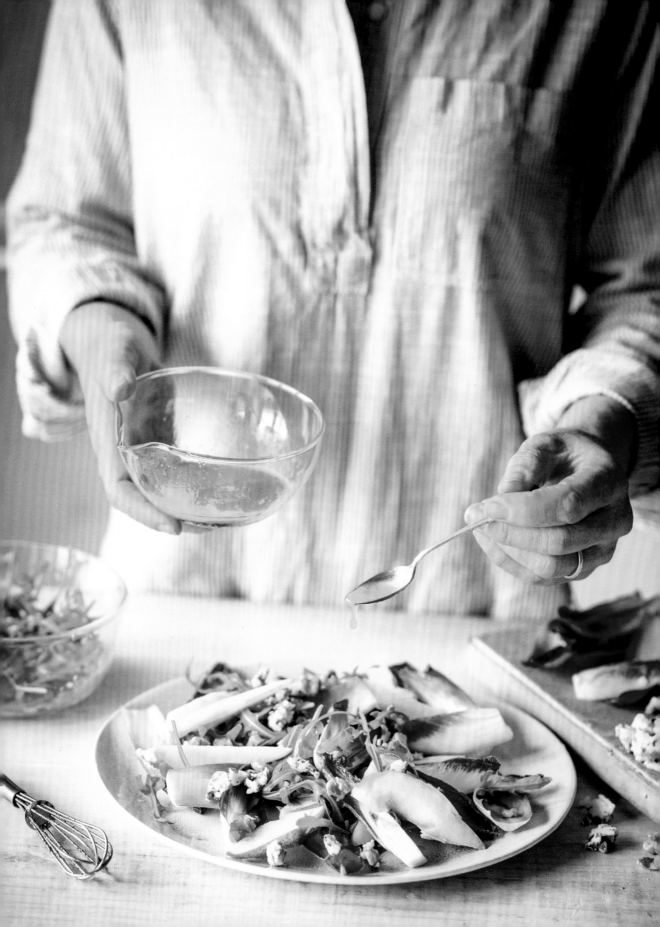

Salads

In this chapter we have included a broad range of salads, from Gut-friendly chicory with blue cheese and walnuts through to the colourful Salmon salad bowl. Enjoy them for lunch or as a light supper. In an ideal world of Med-style living, you'd eat your main meal in the middle of the day and a light meal in the evening – preferably with a brain-boosting siesta thrown in!

Some of the salads are vegetarian – to add more meat or protein, see page 240. Many of them are also suitable for a lunchbox.

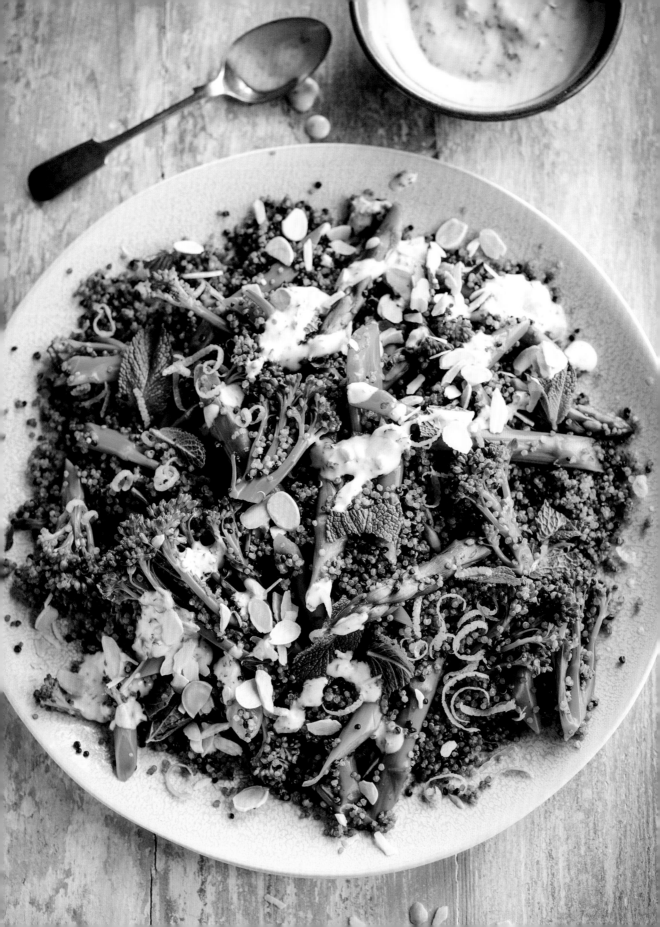

Quinoa, broccoli and asparagus salad

SERVES 2

100g quinoa (ideally a mixture
of white, red and black)
100g long-stemmed
broccoli, trimmed and
each stem cut into three
100g asparagus, trimmed and
each stem cut into three
25g toasted flaked almonds
(see page 18)

For the minted yoghurt dressing
50g full-fat live Greek yoghurt
1 tbsp extra-virgin olive oil
1 tbsp finely chopped fresh mint
finely grated zest and juice
½ lemon
pinch ground cumin

NON-FAST DAYS
Toss cubes of feta into the salad
and add extra almonds.

A filling salad with a gorgeous lemony dressing.
It's also great served alongside grilled meat or fish.
Add extra leaves or other salad-y bits, such as rocket.

1 Third fill a saucepan with water and bring to the boil.
Add the quinoa and cook for 12–15 minutes, or until just
tender, stirring occasionally. The c-shaped husks will start
to float to the surface when the quinoa is ready. Pour the
quinoa into a sieve and rinse under cold running water.
Drain again well, pressing the quinoa in the sieve with the
back of a spoon to remove as much of the water as possible.

2 Meanwhile, bring a second pan of water to the boil and
cook the broccoli and asparagus for 3 minutes. Drain the
asparagus and broccoli and rinse under cold running water.

3 To make the dressing, combine all the ingredients in a
small bowl, adding a little cold water to achieve a pouring
consistency. Season with sea salt and ground black pepper.

4 Place the quinoa, asparagus, broccoli and flaked almonds
in a bowl and toss together well. Season with sea salt and
ground black pepper. Drizzle the dressing over the salad
to serve.

COOK'S TIPS

★ If you have time, griddle the asparagus and broccoli,
instead of blanching, to add a lovely chargrilled flavour.
★ The dressing contains 84cals per tablespoon. Feel free
to add it to a different salad but don't forget to add the
extra calories.

Greek-style salad

SERVES 2

½ cucumber (around 200g),
   halved lengthways and
   thickly sliced
2 ripe medium tomatoes,
   each cut into eight
100g feta, cut into small cubes
½ medium red onion,
   peeled and thinly sliced
50g pitted black olives
   (preferably Kalamata),
   drained
50g mixed salad leaves

For the simple lemon dressing
1 tbsp fresh lemon juice
2 tbsp extra-virgin olive oil

NON-FAST DAYS
Top the salad with roughly
chopped mixed nuts or seeds
and serve with a small
wholemeal pitta bread.

This classic Greek salad works well in a jar or
lidded container, ready to take to work. It can
of course also be assembled in a bowl at home.

1 To make the dressing, whisk the lemon juice, olive
oil, a pinch of sea salt and lots of ground black pepper
in a small bowl to combine. Divide the dressing
between two containers.

2 Divide the cucumber, tomatoes, feta, onion and
olives between the containers and top with the leaves.
The leaves should remain separated from the dressing
at the base of the container until ready to toss.
Pop the lid on and keep chilled until ready to eat.

3 Give the container a shake and eat the salad straight
from the jar, or tip on to a plate to serve.

COOK'S TIPS

★ For added flavour, add a small crushed clove of
garlic and a pinch of mixed dried herbs to the dressing.
★ The dressing contains 66cals per tablespoon. Feel
free to add it to a different salad but don't forget to
add the extra calories.

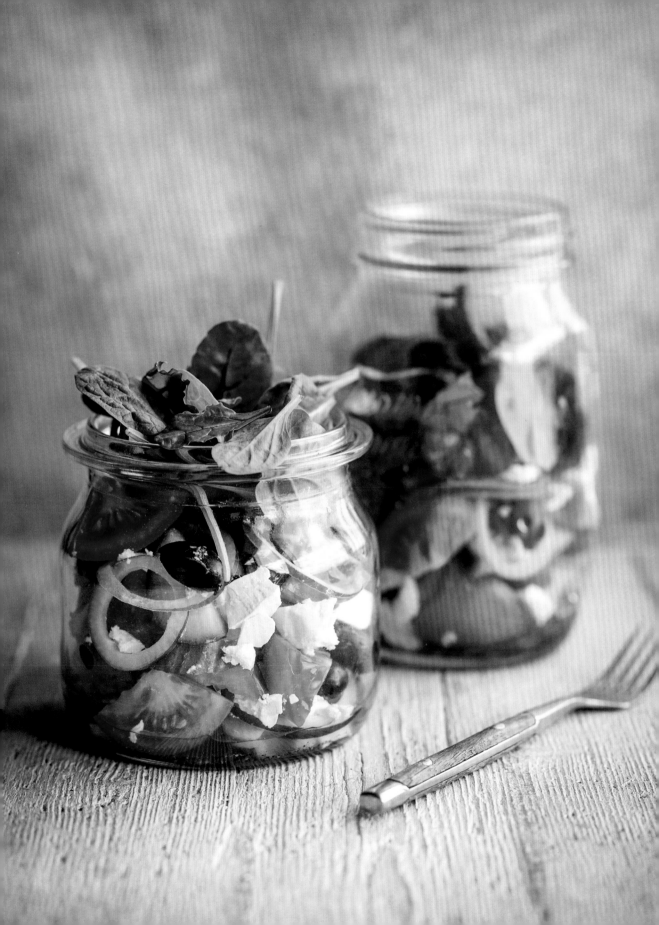

Gut-friendly chicory with blue cheese and walnuts

SERVES 2

20g walnuts, roughly chopped
2 heads chicory, red or white
good handful rocket, or mixed
   rocket, watercress and
   young spinach leaves
1 ripe but firm pear
   (around 125g), quartered,
   cored and sliced
65g soft blue cheese,
   such as Roquefort

For the cider vinegar dressing
1 tbsp live cider vinegar
2 tbsp extra-virgin olive oil

NON-FAST DAYS
Sprinkle the salad with an
extra handful of walnuts and
serve with a couple of thick
slices of warmed wholegrain
bread with olive oil for dipping.
Or you could have this as a
side to another dish.

The chicory and walnuts in this salad contain gut-friendly soluble fibre. Known as a prebiotic, soluble fibre helps the gut bacteria in the colon produce vital nutrients and protects the lining of the gut. This salad makes a good starter, and will help to stimulate the digestion before the main meal.

1 Toast the walnuts in a small frying pan over a medium heat for 2–3 minutes, or until brown in places, shaking the pan occasionally. Tip out on to a board.

2 Trim the chicory and cut 6 thin slices from the root end, then separate the leaves, cutting any that are particularly large in half lengthways. Wash the leaves and drain well.

3 Arrange the chicory in a serving dish and scatter the rocket and pear over the top. Cut the cheese into small pieces and dot on top. Roughly chop the walnuts and sprinkle over the salad.

4 To make the dressing, combine the vinegar and olive oil in a small bowl, season with sea salt and ground black pepper, and whisk until combined. Pour over the salad and toss before serving.

COOK'S TIP

★ The dressing contains 66cals per tablespoon. Feel free to add it to a different salad but don't forget to add the extra calories.

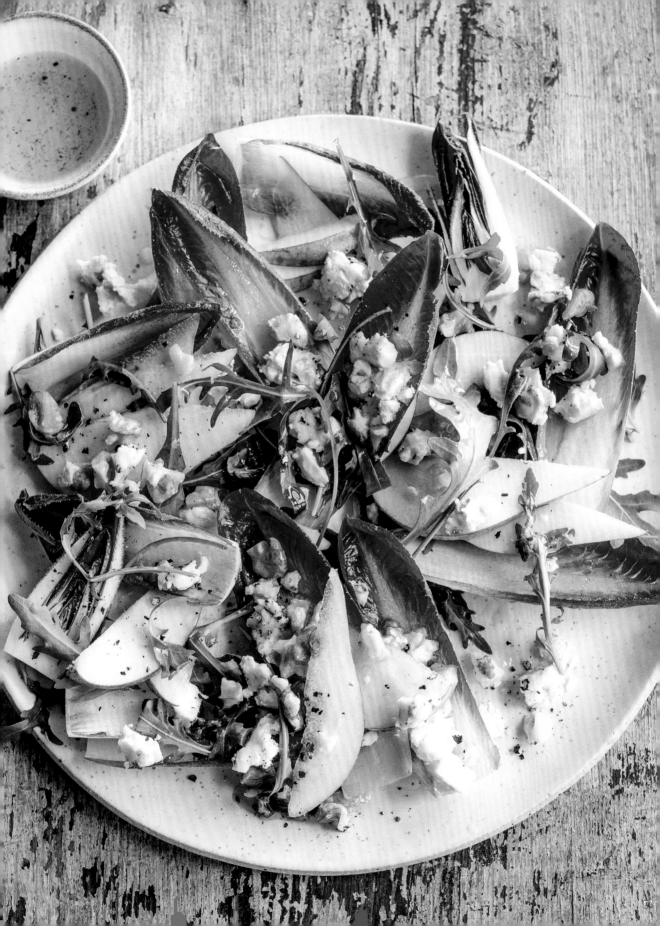

Chicken, bacon and avocado salad

SERVES 2

4 rashers smoked
    streaky bacon
100g mixed salad leaves
8–10 cherry tomatoes, halved
100g cooked chicken
    breast, sliced
1 medium avocado, stoned,
    peeled and sliced
    (see tip on page 40)

For the mustard dressing
2 tbsp extra-virgin olive oil
1 tsp red or white wine vinegar
1 tsp Dijon mustard
1 tsp runny honey

NON-FAST DAYS
Sprinkle the salad with lightly
toasted hazelnuts or a couple
of tablespoons of toasted mixed
seeds. You could toss in a few
tablespoons per person of whole
grains, such as cooked pearl
barley or lentils (available
pre-cooked in packets).

The tiny amount of honey in the dressing here sets
off the saltiness of the bacon perfectly.

1 To make the dressing, whisk the oil with the vinegar,
mustard and honey in a small bowl until slightly thickened.
Season with sea salt and lots of ground black pepper.

2 Place a small non-stick frying pan over a medium heat
and fry the bacon for about 2 minutes on each side, or until
crisp. Transfer to a chopping board and roughly chop.

3 Divide the mixed leaves between two plates. Top with
the tomatoes, sliced chicken, avocado and bacon.

4 Drizzle the mustard dressing over the salad and toss
lightly just before serving.

COOK'S TIPS

★ Buy cooked chicken breast and remove the skin, or
you can roast your own skinless boneless chicken breast.
★ The dressing contains 65cals per tablespoon. Feel free
to add it to a different salad but don't forget to add the
extra calories.

Chicken tikka salad

SERVES 2

2 boneless, skinless chicken
 breasts (each around 175g),
 cut into roughly 3cm chunks
2 tbsp full-fat live
 Greek yoghurt
1 tbsp tikka curry paste
1 tbsp coconut or rapeseed oil
2 Little Gem lettuces, trimmed
 and leaves separated
2 medium tomatoes,
 roughly chopped
½ small red onion, peeled
 and finely chopped
2 tbsp finely chopped fresh
 coriander leaves
fresh mint leaves (optional),
 to serve
lemon or lime wedges,
 to serve

NON-FAST DAYS
Serve with 2–3 tablespoons
of cooked and cooled brown
rice, toasted flaked almonds
and Minty yoghurt raitha
(see page 106).

*A super-tasty chicken salad which makes a great
light lunch.*

1 Place the chicken in a bowl with the yoghurt and tikka
paste. Mix together well, then cover and leave in the fridge
to marinate for at least 1 hour, but ideally several hours
or overnight.

2 Place the oil in a large non-stick frying pan over
a medium–high heat. Add the chicken, season with a
generous pinch of salt and lots of ground black pepper
and fry for 6–8 minutes, turning regularly until lightly
browned and cooked through. Leave to cool if using
for a packed lunch.

3 Divide the lettuce between two wide bowls or lidded
containers.

4 Mix the tomatoes, onion and coriander in a small
bowl and season with sea salt and pepper. Sprinkle over
the lettuce.

5 Arrange the chicken tikka pieces on top, sprinkle with
mint leaves, if using, and serve with lemon or lime wedges
for squeezing over. Keep chilled if not eating straight away.

COOK'S TIP

★ Make sure you use a good-quality tikka paste and not
a curry sauce for the marinade. If you can't get hold of any
paste, use 1 teaspoon hot smoked paprika and 2 teaspoons
medium curry powder instead.

Chicken Caesar-ish salad

SERVES 2

2 Little Gem lettuces, trimmed
   and leaves separated
12 cherry tomatoes, halved
200g cooked chicken breast,
   cut or shredded into
   small pieces
10g mixed seeds
20g Parmesan, finely grated

For the yoghurt dressing
75g full-fat live Greek yoghurt
½ small garlic clove,
   peeled and crushed
pinch dried mixed herbs
1 tbsp extra-virgin olive oil

NON-FAST DAYS
Increase the portion size
and add extra seeds.

The mixed seeds here add the crunch usually provided by croutons and are far more nutritious.

1 To make the dressing, combine the yoghurt, garlic, herbs, oil and 2 tablespoons cold water in a bowl and mix well. Season with a pinch of sea salt and lots of ground black pepper.

2 Wash the lettuce and drain well. Divide the leaves between two shallow bowls or lidded containers and scatter with the tomatoes.

3 Place the chicken on top, sprinkle with the mixed seeds and Parmesan and drizzle with the dressing. Season with ground black pepper and serve.

COOK'S TIPS

★ If taking as a packed lunch, put the dressing in a small lidded pot and drizzle over the salad just before serving. Keep the salad and dressing chilled until needed.
★ The dressing contains 34cals per tablespoon. Feel free to add it to a different salad but don't forget to add the extra calories.

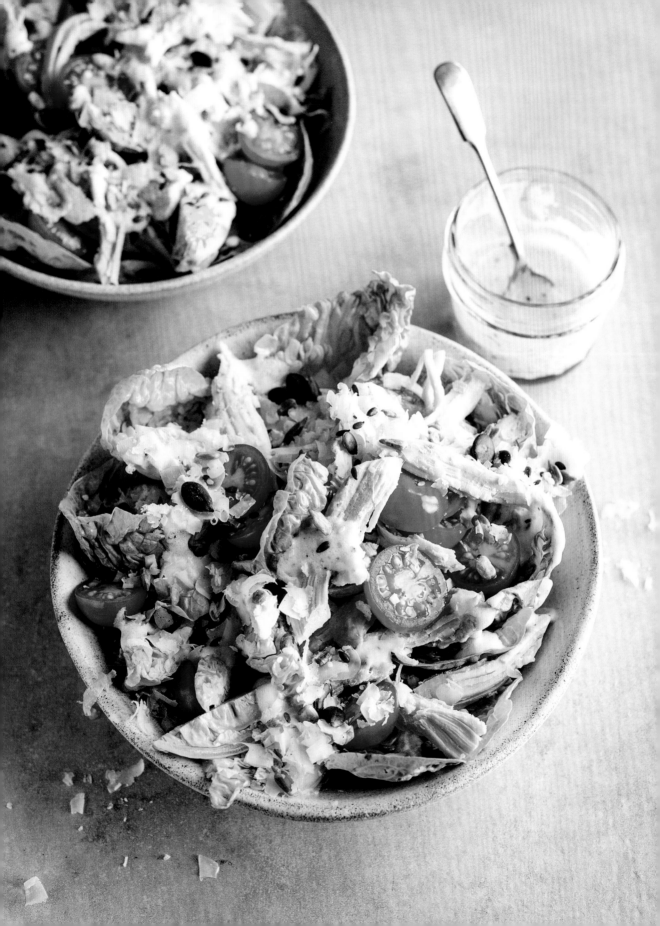

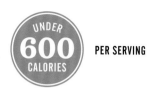
Salmon salad bowl

SERVES 2

25g wholegrain brown rice,
    or brown and wild rice mix
75g frozen edamame beans
    or frozen peas
2 × 120g salmon fillets
1 tsp sesame seeds
pinch crushed dried chilli
    flakes (optional)
2 large handfuls young
    spinach leaves or mixed
    baby salad leaves
½ medium avocado, stoned,
    peeled and chopped
    (see tip on page 40)
1 medium carrot, trimmed
    and coarsely grated
2 spring onions, trimmed
    and finely sliced
4 radishes, trimmed and sliced
lime wedges, to serve

For the soy and lime dressing
2 tbsp dark soy sauce
1 tbsp sesame oil
1 tsp fresh lime juice
1 tsp runny honey

NON-FAST DAYS
Choose larger fillets – you will
need to cook them a few minutes
longer. Increase the quantity
of rice, or cook diced butternut
squash alongside the salmon
(roast for 10 minutes more).

Serve the salad warm as a delicious lunch or supper,
or take it to work in a lidded container for a nutritious
and filling packed lunch.

1 Preheat the oven to 200°C/fan 180°C/Gas 6 and line
a small baking tray with foil.

2 Half fill a small saucepan with water and bring to the
boil. Add the rice and cook for about 20 minutes, or until
tender. Add the edamame beans or peas and return to
the boil, stirring. Drain immediately.

3 To make the dressing, combine the soy sauce, sesame
oil, lime juice and honey in a small bowl and whisk well.

4 Place the salmon, skin-side down, on the prepared
tray and drizzle with 2 teaspoons of the dressing. Sprinkle
with the sesame seeds and chilli flakes, if using. Bake
for 10–12 minutes, or until just cooked. (It is ready
when the salmon flakes into large pieces easily when
prodded with a fork.)

5 Divide the leaves, rice and beans or peas between two
bowls. Add the leaves and arrange the avocado, carrot,
spring onions and radishes alongside. Flake the salmon
into the bowl (leaving behind the skin), drizzle with the
rest of the dressing and serve with lime wedges for
squeezing over.

COOK'S TIPS

★ Make the full amount, even if you only need one serving,
as the rest will keep well in the fridge for the next day.
★ The dressing contains 39cals per tablespoon – without
the honey. Feel free to add it to a different salad but don't
forget to add the extra calories.

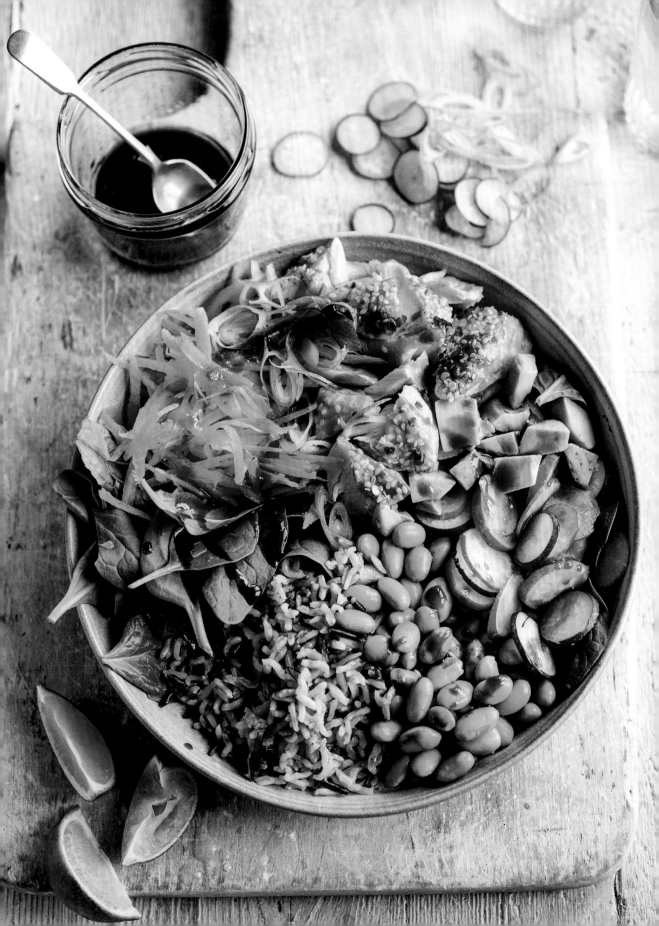

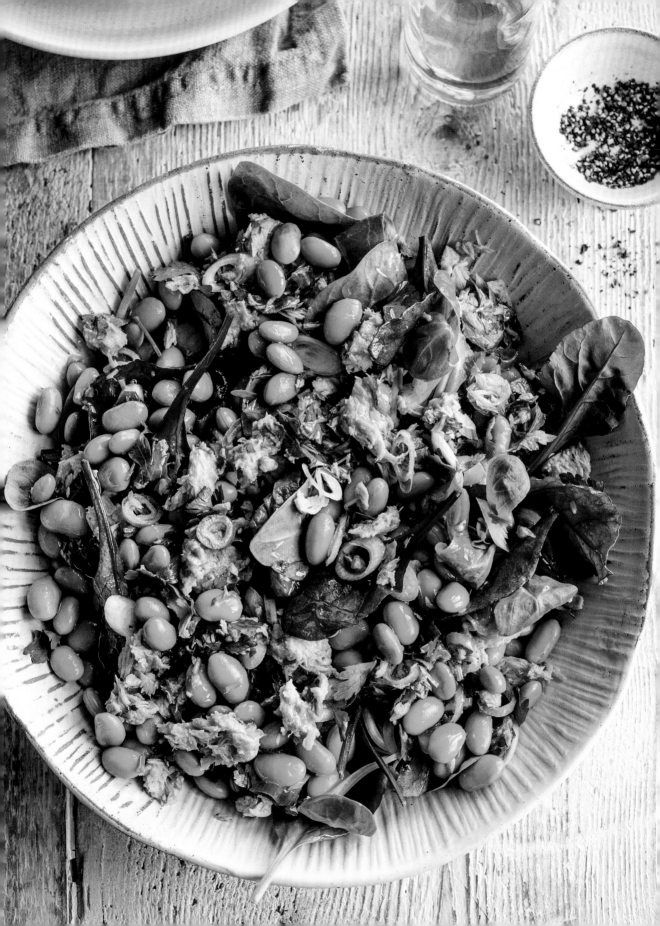

Edamame and tuna salad

SERVES 2

200g frozen edamame beans

2 spring onions, trimmed
and thinly sliced

1 × 110g can no-drain tuna
steak in olive oil

15g fresh flat-leaf parsley
or coriander, leaves
roughly chopped

1½ tbsp live cider vinegar

3 tbsp extra-virgin olive oil

2 large handfuls rocket
or mixed leaves

NON-FAST DAYS
Increase the portion size and
stir in a few tablespoonfuls
per person of cooked whole
grains, such as quinoa or pearl
barley (available pre-cooked
in packets).

Protein- and fibre-rich edamame beans make a great
addition to any salad. These versatile young beans
have a fresh, green crunch to them and make this
a wonderfully filling salad.

1 Tip the edamame beans into a heatproof bowl and
cover with just-boiled water from a kettle. Stir and leave
for 1 minute to allow the beans to thaw (there's no need
to cook them). Drain and rinse under cold water.

2 Place the beans, spring onions, tuna and herbs
in a bowl and use a fork a break the tuna into flakes.
Drizzle the vinegar and olive oil over the salad, season
with sea salt and lots of ground black pepper and toss
together well.

3 Fold in the leaves just before serving.

COOK'S TIPS

★ Cans of tuna come in different sizes and some don't
need draining. As long as you end up with around 110g
tuna (drained weight) the calories will remain similar.
★ Add a square of dried nori seaweed, cut into little pieces,
for extra flavour and an omega-3 boost, and scatter over
a pinch of crushed dried chilli flakes if you like a bit
more bite.

Crab, courgette and avocado salad

SERVES 2

20g pine nuts

2 medium courgettes (each around 250g), trimmed

1 small avocado, stoned, peeled and diced (see tip on page 40)

2 large handfuls rocket

100g white crabmeat, tinned or fresh

1 red chilli, thinly sliced or diced (optional)

For the lime dressing

3 tbsp extra-virgin olive oil

1 tbsp fresh lime juice

½ tsp wholegrain mustard

1 tbsp finely chopped fresh mint

NON-FAST DAYS
Serve with warm wholegrain bread and olive oil for dipping.

Michael and I both lived by the sea as children and love all seafood. This super summer salad is very healthy and also contains minerals that we can be lacking, such as selenium and iodine.

1 To make the dressing, combine the olive oil, lime juice, mustard and mint in a small bowl and whisk together well.

2 Scatter the pine nuts into a small frying pan and toast over a medium heat for 1–2 minutes, stirring frequently, until lightly browned. Tip on to a plate and set aside.

3 Slice the courgettes into long, wide strips using a vegetable peeler and place in a wide bowl. Add the avocado and rocket leaves, season with sea salt and ground black pepper and toss lightly.

4 Scatter the crabmeat on top and sprinkle with the pine nuts and chilli, if using. Drizzle with the dressing to serve.

COOK'S TIPS

★ You can find hand-picked crabmeat sold in small pots at the fishmonger or supermarket.

★ The dressing contains 75cals per tablespoon. Feel free to add it to a different salad but don't forget to add the extra calories.

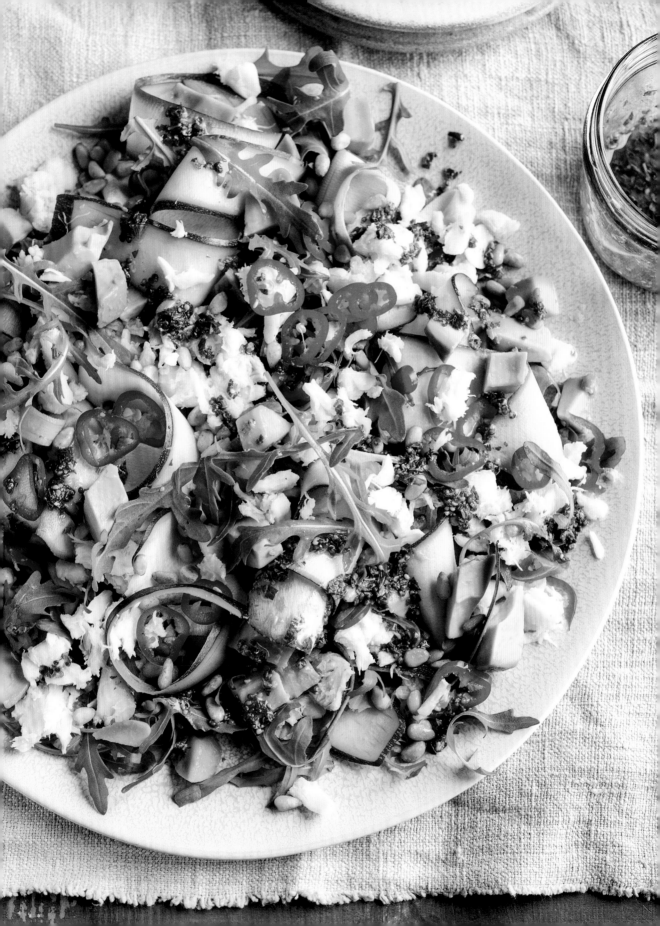

Tuna Niçoise salad

SERVES 2

100g green beans,
   trimmed and halved
100g cauliflower,
   cut into small florets
2 medium eggs, fridge cold
50g mixed salad leaves
8 cherry tomatoes, halved
1 × 110g can no-drain tuna
   steak in olive oil
30g canned anchovies
   in oil, drained
40g pitted black or
   green olives

*For the creamy garlicky
yoghurt dressing*
1 tbsp extra-virgin olive oil
50g full-fat live Greek yoghurt
½ small garlic clove,
   peeled and crushed

NON-FAST DAYS
Increase the portion size.

A classic salad with a low-carb twist, in which
cauliflower takes the place of the traditional potatoes.

1 To make the dressing, combine the oil, yoghurt, garlic
and 2 tablespoons cold water in a small bowl and mix
well. Season with a pinch of sea salt and some ground
black pepper.

2 Half fill a small pan with water and bring to the boil.
Add the beans and cauliflower florets, return to the boil
and cook for 3 minutes. Lift out with a slotted spoon
and plunge into a bowl of cold water.

3 Return the water to the boil. Add the eggs and cook for
8 minutes. Lift out with a slotted spoon and plunge into
a separate bowl of very cold water.

4 Drain the green beans and cauliflower well, then arrange
them on two plates with the mixed leaves and tomatoes.

5 Peel the eggs, cut into quarters and place on the salad
with flakes of tuna, the anchovies and olives.

6 Drizzle with the dressing just before serving.

COOK'S TIPS

★ If you aren't using fridge-cold eggs, decrease the cooking
time by a minute or two.
★ The dressing contains 41cals per tablespoon. Feel free
to add it to a different salad but don't forget to add the
extra calories.

Homemade coleslaw

SERVES 4

100g full-fat live yoghurt, ideally Greek

100g good-quality mayonnaise

¼ medium red cabbage (around 200g)

1 medium carrot, trimmed and coarsely grated into long, thin shreds

2 spring onions, trimmed and finely sliced

1 celery stick, trimmed and thinly sliced (optional)

5:2

NON-FAST DAYS
Increase the portion size or serve with a small wholemeal pitta.

A crisp and colourful salad that makes a fibre-rich addition to any meal.

1 Mix the yoghurt, mayonnaise and 2 tablespoons cold water in a large bowl with a little black pepper.

2 Remove any damaged outer leaves from the cabbage and cut out the tough central core. Shred the cabbage as finely as possible and add to the yoghurt dressing.

3 Add the carrot, spring onions and celery, if using, to the bowl and toss everything together well.

COOK'S TIP

★ You can also serve this as a light meal for two, if you add 50g chopped nuts (74cals a serving), 100g shredded cooked chicken (44cals a serving) or 100g sliced ham (127cals a serving).

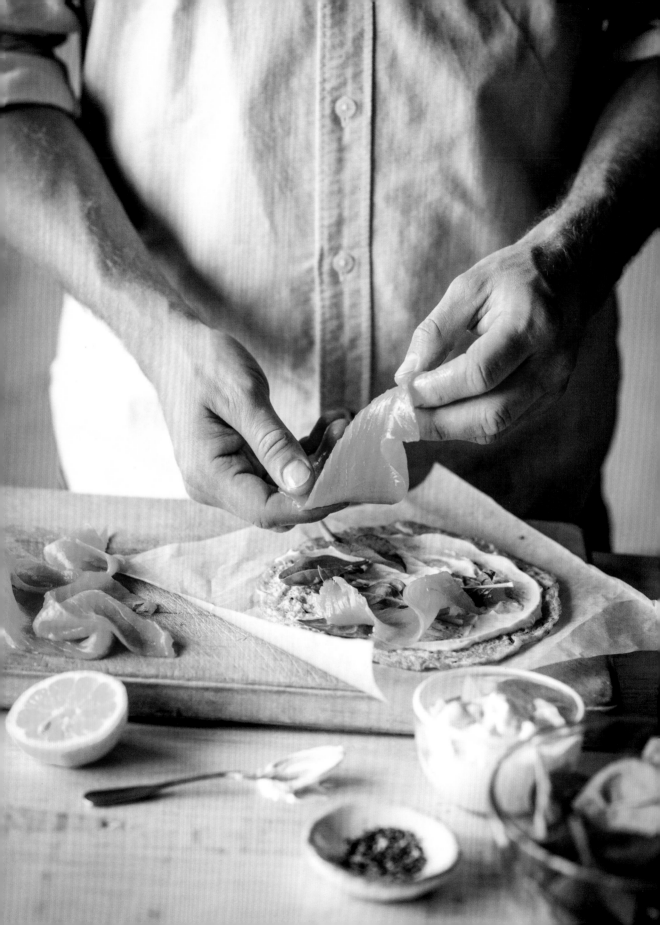

Food on the Move

For those who work in offices, or are doing shift work or travelling, eating healthily can be a challenge. This chapter is partly about anticipation and preparation, so all the recipes are easy to assemble in advance. With instant, tasty meals that keep you feeling full and satisfied, even on a fast day, you will be much less likely to reach for something sweet, starchy and processed on the hoof, however tempting!

Note: most lunch boxes need a cold pack or to be kept in a fridge. These recipes can work as portable breakfasts, too.

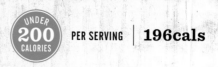
Lettuce wraps – three ways

Make lettuce your new 'bread' when you have a sandwich. Many people munch on starchy sandwiches for at least one meal a day. Much better to dump the bread and just eat the filling. If you need to eat on the go, simply wrap your lettuce wraps in foil to hold them together.

SERVES 2

1 romaine lettuce heart

1 Remove the large outer leaves and set aside 6–8 of them to provide the cups. Slice the smaller leaves and place in a medium bowl.

2 Add the rest of the ingredients to the bowl, season with sea salt and ground black pepper and mix well.

3 Spoon the filling into the wraps and serve.

COOK'S TIPS

★ If preparing for one person, keep the remaining filling in the fridge to assemble the following day.
★ If you can't get hold of the piquanté peppers for the **Mediterranean tuna lettuce wrap**, use any roasted peppers from a jar and add a pinch of chilli flakes.

Mediterranean tuna

1 × 110g can no-drain tuna steak
   in olive oil
½ small red onion, peeled
   and very finely sliced
20g small Peppadew piquanté peppers
   from a jar, drained and sliced
10 cherry tomatoes, quartered
40g black or green pitted olives,
   drained and halved
1 tbsp extra-virgin olive oil

NON-FAST DAYS
Add chopped avocado to the salad mix, or double the portion size.

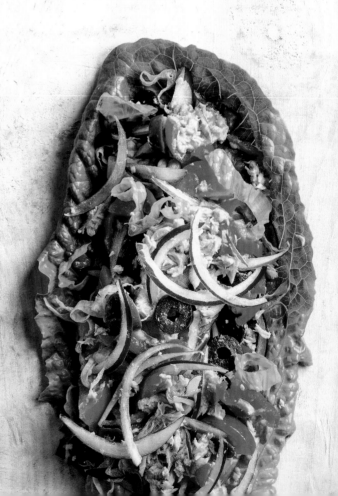

UNDER **200** CALORIES | PER SERVING | **143cals**

Prawn mayo

100g cooked and peeled prawns,
   thawed if frozen
25g good-quality mayonnaise
2 tsp reduced sugar tomato ketchup
8 cherry tomatoes, quartered
¼ cucumber (around 100g),
   cut into roughly 1cm chunks

5:2

NON-FAST DAYS
Double the portion size.

 UNDER **400** CALORIES | PER SERVING | **308cals**

Pesto bean salad

½ × 400g can mixed beans,
   drained and rinsed
¼ small red onion, peeled
   and finely chopped
50g roasted peppers from a jar,
   drained and chopped
125g ball mozzarella, drained,
   halved and torn
2 tbsp fresh basil pesto

5:2

NON-FAST DAYS
Add a drizzle of extra-virgin olive oil and
some chopped avocado to the salad mix.

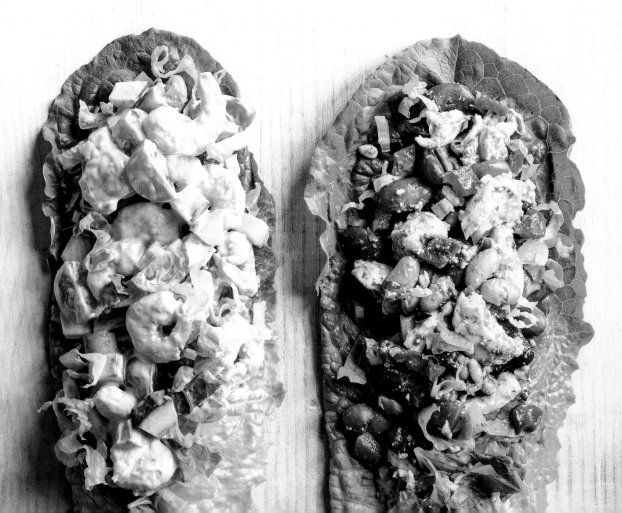

PER SERVING | **318cals** | PROTEIN **12g** | FAT **16.5g** | FIBRE **3.5g** | CARBS **29g**

Nori tuna wraps

SERVES 2
1 × 60g can no-drain
  tuna in olive oil
1 tbsp good-quality
  mayonnaise
1 tbsp fresh lime juice
2 sheets dried nori, each
  around 20cm square
½ medium avocado, stoned,
  peeled and mashed
  (see tip page 40)
150g cooked and cooled
  brown rice
25g cucumber, cut into
  long thin batons

For the dip
2 tbsp dark soy sauce
¼ tsp crushed dried
  chilli flakes

5:2

NON-FAST DAYS
Increase the portion size.

This delicious, sushi-style seaweed wrap gives you the best marine-based omega-3 oils and iodine you can find and is surprisingly easy to make. Nori, a type of dried seaweed, is often sold in square sheets; you'll find it in the Japanese or World Food section of larger supermarkets and specialist stores.

1 Mash the tuna with the mayonnaise, lime juice and a good grinding of black pepper in a small bowl.

2 Place one of the nori sheets on a board, shiny side down, and spread half of the mashed avocado almost all the way over it. Top with half the rice and press it down lightly with the back of a spoon.

3 Spoon half the tuna mixture in a line across the centre of the rice and place the cucumber sticks beside it, all lying in the same direction.

4 Roll the nori firmly around the filling, using two hands. Trim the edges then cut into six pieces. Repeat with the remaining nori and filling.

5 To make the dip, mix the soy sauce with the chilli flakes and serve alongside.

COOK'S TIP

★ If taking to work, wrap unsliced in cling film or foil.

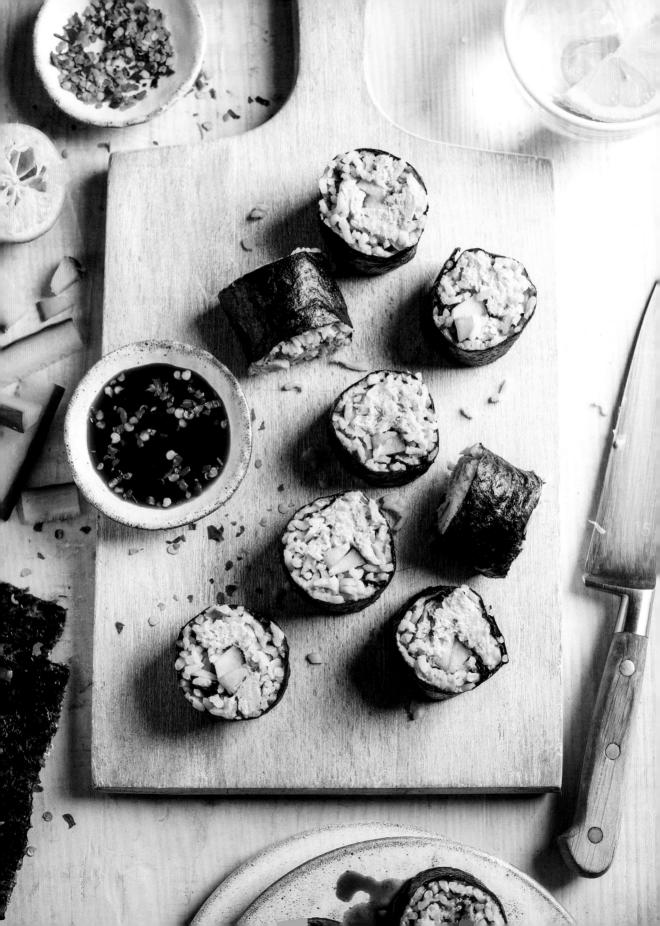

Low-carb omelette wraps

A handy sandwich alternative that can be made the night before, ready to take to work. Make your wrap as follows, and spread with one of the fillings opposite.

SERVES 1

1 large egg
½ tsp olive or rapeseed oil

1 Beat the egg in a small bowl until smooth. Season with ground black pepper.

2 Brush a non-stick frying pan (base no larger than around 19cm) with the oil and place over a medium heat.

3 Pour the egg into the pan and swirl so that it spreads around to completely cover the base. Cook for 1–2 minutes or until set.

4 Loosen with a spatula then flip and cook for 10 seconds more. Turn out on to a board and leave to cool for a few minutes.

COOK'S TIPS

★ If you don't have a small frying pan, use a larger one and double the quantities. Cut the wrap in half to serve two people, or chill and save the second half for the next day.
★ If taking to work, roll your wrap tightly in foil and refrigerate in a lidded container.

NON-FAST DAYS
Have two!

Smoked salmon and cream cheese

15g medium-fat soft cheese (around 1 tbsp),
such as Philadelphia
50g smoked salmon (around 2 slices)
small handful mixed salad leaves
or young spinach leaves

1 Spread the egg wrap with the soft cheese, season with ground black pepper and top with the smoked salmon and leaves.

2 Roll up firmly and cut in half diagonally to serve.

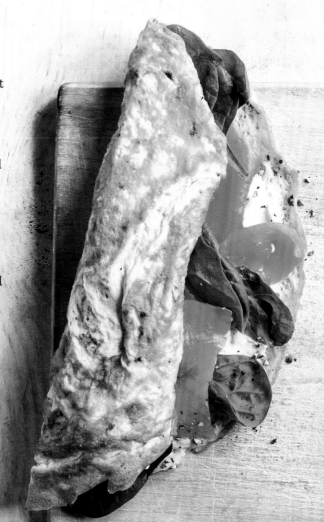

Ham, cheese and herb

1 tsp good-quality mayonnaise
1 thin slice smoked ham (around 20g)
15g mature Cheddar, finely grated
2 roasted red peppers from a jar
   (around 50g), drained and sliced
small handful mixed salad leaves

1 Spread the egg wrap thinly with mayonnaise, season with ground black pepper, then top with the ham, grated cheese, peppers and leaves.

2 Roll up firmly and cut in half diagonally to serve.

Hummus, carrot and spinach

30g olive oil hummus (around 2 tbsp)
1 small carrot, trimmed and coarsely grated
small handful young spinach leaves

1 Spread the egg wrap with the hummus, season with sea salt and ground black pepper and top with the grated carrot and spinach.

2 Roll up firmly and cut in half diagonally to serve.

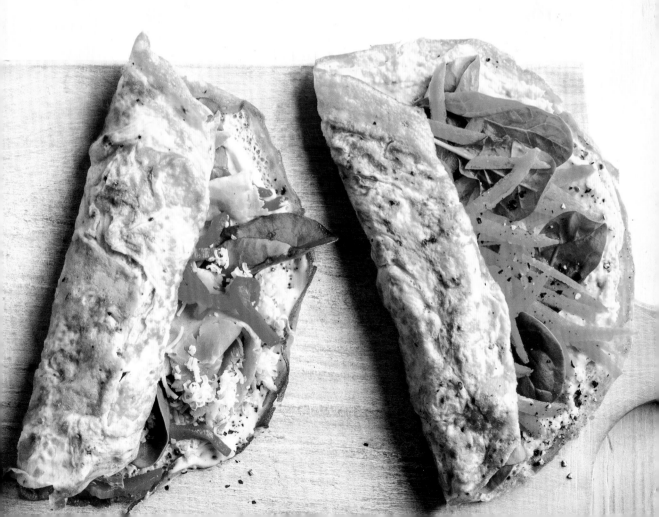

Super-speedy portable lunch

Two easy lunch ideas that you should be able to make from the store cupboard at home. Serve with wholegrain, rye or sourdough crispbreads, if you like, but remember to add the extra calories.

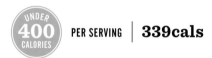 PER SERVING | **339cals**

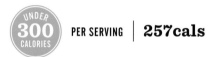 PER SERVING | **257cals**

Sardines and beetroot

SERVES 1

1 × 120g can sardines in olive oil
5 slices beetroot in vinegar from a jar
   (about 50g), drained and roughly chopped
1 tbsp good-quality mayonnaise

1 Drain and mash the sardines in
a small bowl.

2 Add all the remaining ingredients to the
bowl and mix well. Season with sea salt
and a grinding of black pepper to taste.

Tuna and sweetcorn

SERVES 1

1 × 60g can no-drain tuna in oil
½ × 198g can sweetcorn, drained
1 tbsp good-quality mayonnaise
1 dill cucumber (gherkin), chopped

1 Mix all the ingredients together in
a small bowl. Season with sea salt and
a grinding of black pepper to taste.

Mike's peppered mackerel paté

SERVES 4

3 peppered smoked mackerel fillets (around 270g), skinned and flaked

150g medium-fat soft cheese, such as Philadelphia

finely grated zest and juice ½ small lemon

assorted vegetable sticks (such as celery, carrots and courgettes) or cauliflower florets, to serve

5:2

NON-FAST DAYS
Serve with seeded crackers or spread on dark rye bread fingers.

I remember Michael making a version of this at medical school, simply mashed together in two minutes – delicious. It keeps well in the fridge for up to three days.

1 Put the mackerel, soft cheese, lemon zest and juice and lots of ground black pepper in a bowl. Mash vigorously with a fork. Alternatively, for a smoother texture, use a stick blender or blitz in a food processor on the pulse setting.

2 Adjust the seasoning to taste, spoon into a small dish and serve with the crudité vegetables; or spread on to slices of courgette and serve as low-carb 'blinis'. (Don't worry about the calories in the crudité.)

COOK'S TIPS

★ For an extra kick, add a few drops of Tabasco to the paté.
★ You can use plain smoked mackerel fillets if you prefer.

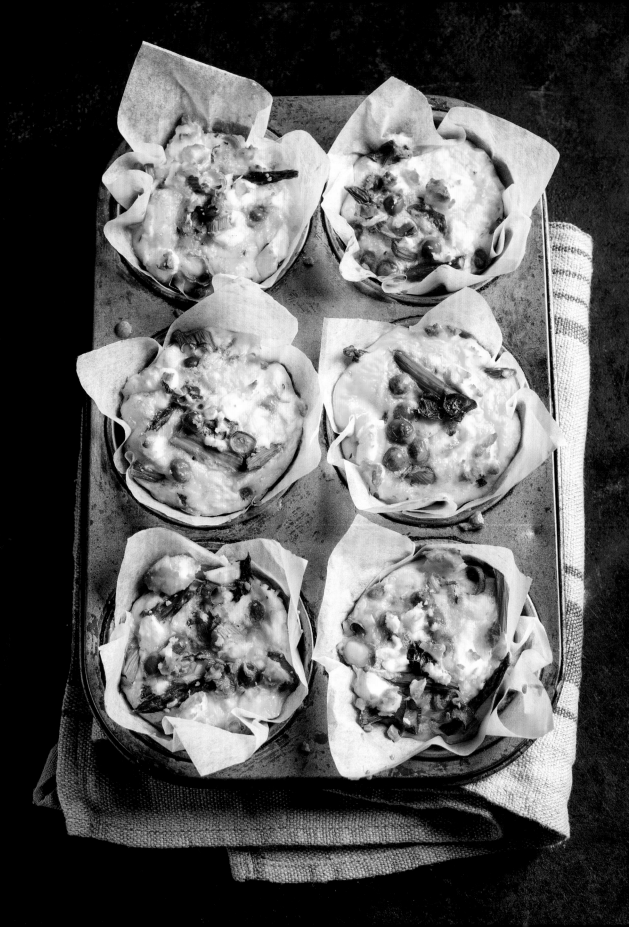

UNDER **200** CALORIES

Asparagus, pea and mint frittata muffins

SERVES 6
2 tsp olive or rapeseed oil
150g slender asparagus, trimmed and each stem cut into 2–3cm pieces
100g frozen peas
4 spring onions, trimmed and thinly sliced
3–4 tbsp finely chopped fresh mint
6 large eggs
65g feta, broken into small chunks

NON-FAST DAYS
Enjoy an extra muffin and add a dressing to the salad you serve alongside. You might also scatter the salad with toasted seeds.

A lovely portable lunch. Serve warm or cold with a generous salad or freshly cooked greens.

1 Preheat the oven to 200°C/fan 180°C/Gas 6 and generously oil a deep, 6-hole muffin tin. Cut six pieces of non-stick baking paper (roughly 10cm squared) and use to line the tins, leaving the excess peaking over the sides.

2 Third fill a large pan with water and bring to the boil. Add the asparagus and cook for 4 minutes. Add the peas and cook for 1 minute more. Drain the vegetables well and tip into a large bowl with the spring onions and mint.

3 Beat the eggs in a separate bowl with a good pinch of sea salt and lots of ground black pepper.

4 Divide the vegetables between the six muffin cases and top with the chunks of feta.

5 Pour the egg over the vegetables then bake in the preheated oven for about 20 minutes, or until puffed up and light golden brown.

COOK'S TIP

★ Choose young asparagus that isn't too thick – if you do end up with thicker stems, cut them in half lengthways before slicing.

| PER SERVING | **294cals** | PROTEIN **22g** | FAT **20g** | FIBRE **2g** | CARBS **5g**

Goat's cheese frittata

SERVES 4

1 tbsp olive oil, plus
    extra for greasing
1 medium red onion, peeled
    and finely chopped
1 red pepper, deseeded and cut
    into roughly 1.5cm chunks
1 medium courgette, trimmed
    and cut into roughly
    1.5cm chunks
100g goat's cheese,
    cut into small chunks
8 medium eggs

NON-FAST DAYS
Enjoy a larger portion.

Great for lunchboxes but also brilliant served warm with a crunchy green and red salad, or cooked green vegetables, as a light meal at home.

1 Preheat the oven to 200°C/fan 180°C/Gas 6. Grease and line the base of a 20cm square cake tin (not loose-based) with non-stick baking paper.

2 Heat the oil in a large non-stick frying pan and gently fry the onion, pepper and courgette for 5 minutes, or until softened. Tip into the prepared tin and spread to the sides. Scatter the goat's cheese over the vegetables.

3 Whisk the eggs in a small bowl with sea salt and lots of ground black pepper until thoroughly combined.

4 Pour over the cheese and vegetables and bake in the preheated oven for 20 minutes, or until the frittata has set and is slightly puffy and golden brown.

5 Cut into squares or bars to serve.

COOK'S TIP

★ You can also use a shallow ovenproof dish for this recipe – an 18–20cm ceramic quiche dish would work well – but you will need to cook it for a little longer.

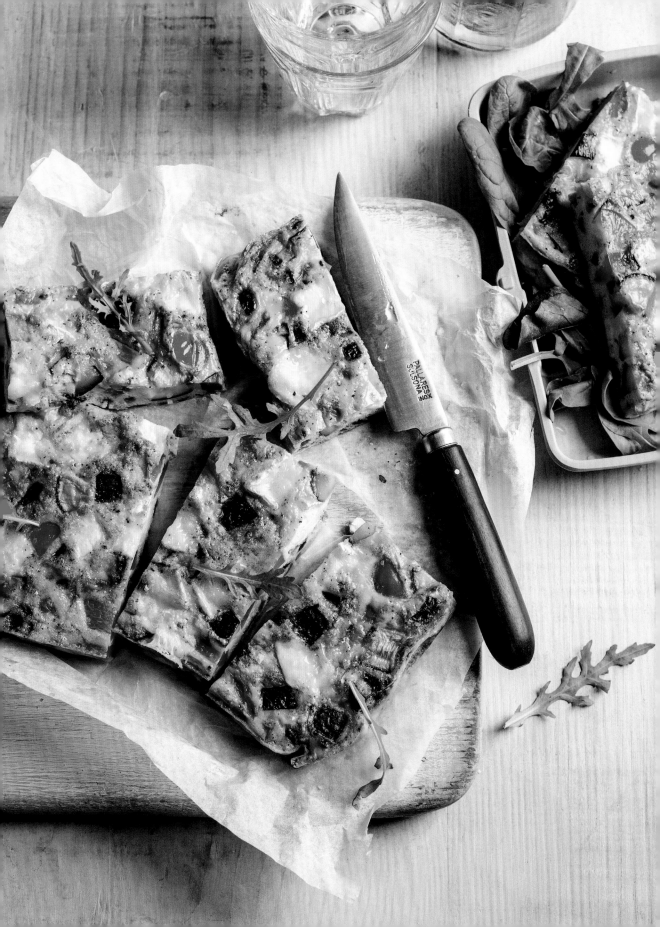

PER SERVING | **228cals** | PROTEIN **15.5g** | FAT **14.5g** | FIBRE **5g** | CARBS **6g**

Celeriac Spanish omelette

SERVES 4

300g celeriac, peeled
   and cut into roughly
   2cm chunks
1 tbsp olive oil
1 medium onion, peeled
   and finely chopped
2 small peppers
   (1 red and 1 yellow),
   deseeded and thinly sliced
40g chorizo, finely chopped
10g bunch flat-leaf parsley,
   leaves finely chopped
6 medium eggs, beaten

5:2

NON-FAST DAYS
Add a dressing to the salad,
if serving one alongside,
and serve larger portions
of the omelette.

Making a Spanish omelette with celeriac rather than potatoes reduces the starchy carbs and adds a delicious subtle flavour. Serve warm or cold with a large salad.

1 Third fill a saucepan with water and bring to the boil. Add the celeriac, return to the boil and cook for 5 minutes. Drain well.

2 Heat the oil in an ovenproof non-stick frying pan (with a base roughly 19cm diameter). Add the onion and peppers and cook over a medium heat for 5 minutes, or until softened and beginning to colour.

3 Add the chorizo and celeriac, season well with sea salt and plenty of ground black pepper and cook for a further 3 minutes, stirring.

4 Stir the parsley into the eggs, then pour over the vegetables. Reduce the heat and cook for 5 minutes without stirring. Meanwhile, preheat the grill to a medium-hot setting.

5 Place the frying pan under the grill and cook for a further 4–5 minutes, or until the eggs are set, then remove and leave to stand for 5 minutes. Turn out on to a board, cut into quarters and serve.

COOK'S TIPS

★ If you don't have a suitable pan, tip the lightly fried vegetables into a quiche dish, add the egg and parsley and bake in the oven until set instead.
★ You can store leftover portions in the fridge, covered, for a couple of days, or take it to work for lunch.
★ For a vegetarian version, simply leave out the chorizo and reduce the calories by 48cals per serving.

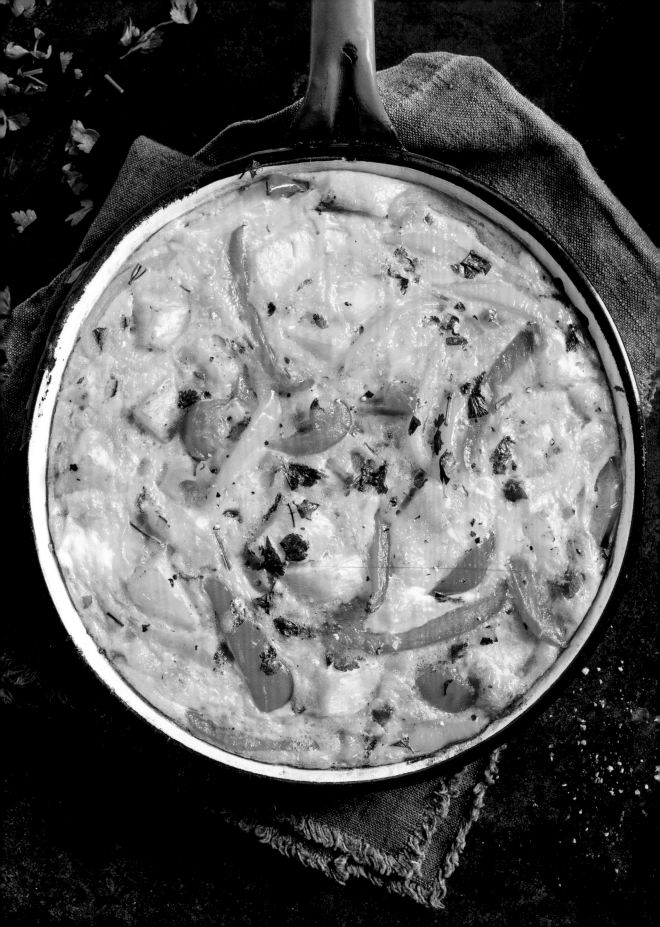

Pesto beans with Parma ham

SERVES 2

80g mixed baby leaf salad

1 × 400g can cannellini beans, drained and rinsed

1 tbsp fresh basil pesto

15g mixed nuts, roughly chopped

10g Parmesan, shavings or freshly grated

4 thin slices Parma ham or prosciutto

1 tbsp extra-virgin olive oil

NON-FAST DAYS

Serve with wholegrain bread and drizzle with more olive oil.

A fab, instant and filling lunch which also works well in a lunch box.

1 Scatter the leaves on to two plates or into two lidded containers.

2 Mix the cannellini beans with the pesto then divide between the plates or containers.

3 Scatter the nuts and Parmesan over the beans, top with the ham, then drizzle with the oil. Finally, season with ground black pepper and serve.

Fast falafel, hummus and beetroot salad

SERVES 1

40g mixed salad leaves

2 ready-made falafel (around 50g)

30g olive oil hummus (around 2 tbsp)

30g ready-made tzatziki (around 2 tbsp)

1 small cooked beetroot (around 40g), drained and quartered

1 tbsp extra-virgin olive oil

1 tsp mixed seeds

Pick up these ready-prepared ingredients in the supermarket to make your own delicious instant salad bowl.

1 Place the leaves in a bowl or lidded container.

2 Add the falafel, hummus, tzatziki and beetroot pieces.

3 Drizzle over the oil, sprinkle with the mixed seeds and serve.

NON-FAST DAYS

Enjoy with a small wholemeal pitta bread.

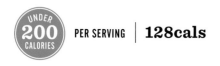

UNDER 200 CALORIES | PER SERVING | **128cals**

UNDER 100 CALORIES | PER SERVING | **59cals**

Celeriac skordalia

An indulgent Greek dip made with celeriac and almonds instead of potatoes and bread. Serve with veg sticks.

SERVES 6
½ medium celeriac (around 300g),
    peeled and cut into roughly 3cm chunks
6 garlic cloves, peeled
50g ground almonds
2 tbsp fresh lemon juice
½ tsp flaked sea salt
50ml extra-virgin olive oil
handful freshly chopped parsley, to serve

1 Third fill a saucepan with water and bring to the boil. Add the celeriac and garlic, return to the boil and cook for 15 minutes, or until the celeriac is very tender. Drain over a bowl and reserve the cooking water.

2 Place the celeriac and garlic in a food processor, add 1 ladleful (around 100ml) of the cooking water and blitz to a purée. Add the ground almonds, lemon juice and salt, season with ground black pepper and blitz.

3 Keep the motor running and add the olive oil in a thin stream, reserving about 1 teaspoon for serving. Blend until the purée thickens and becomes smooth.

4 Transfer to a small bowl, drizzle with the reserved olive oil, sprinkle with fresh parsley and serve.

NON-FAST DAYS
Serve with fingers of toasted wholemeal pitta bread.

Minty yoghurt raitha

Serve as a cooling accompaniment to curries, or as a dip with veg sticks.

SERVES 4
⅓ cucumber (around 135g)
150g full-fat live Greek yoghurt
3–4 tbsp finely chopped fresh mint

1 Cut the cucumber in half lengthways and scoop out the seeds with a teaspoon. Coarsely grate the flesh on to a board then transfer to a bowl.

2 Add the yoghurt and mint, and season with a good pinch of sea salt and lots of ground black pepper. Mix well and leave for 20–30 minutes to allow the flavours to mingle.

3 Keep chilled until ready to serve.

COOK'S TIP

★ If using as a dip, add 1 green chilli, deseeded and finely chopped, for a bit more zing.

NON-FAST DAYS
Serve with fingers of toasted wholemeal pitta bread or wholegrain seeded crackers.

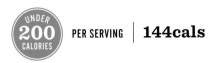

PER SERVING | **144cals**

PER SERVING | **88cals**

Minted beetroot hummus

A magnificent magenta-coloured hummus. Beetroot is surprisingly low in calories but high in nutrients. It can help reduce blood pressure and inflammation.

SERVES 6

300g cooked beetroot, drained and quartered
1 × 400g can chickpeas, drained and rinsed
1 garlic clove, peeled and halved
1 tsp ground coriander
2 tbsp finely chopped fresh mint leaves
2 tbsp extra-virgin olive oil
2 tbsp fresh lemon juice
½ tsp flaked sea salt
2 tbsp mixed seeds, toasted (see page 243)

1 Put all the ingredients, except the seeds, in a food processor and season with ground black pepper. Blitz until almost smooth. Adjust the seasoning and lightly blitz again. Spoon into a bowl.

2 Toast the mixed seeds in a small dry frying pan over a low heat for about 2 minutes, shaking the pan regularly. Sprinkle over the hummus to serve.

COOK'S TIP

★ Keep covered in the fridge for up to 3 days or you can freeze for up to 1 month.

NON-FAST DAYS
Drizzle with olive oil and top with an extra sprinkling of toasted mixed seeds. Serve with fingers of toasted wholemeal pitta bread or wholemeal crispbread (see tip page 238).

Roasted red pepper hummus

A great way to use up a jar of roasted red peppers. Serve with non-starchy veg crudités.

SERVES 6

175g roasted red peppers, from a jar, drained
1 × 400g can chickpeas, drained and rinsed
1 garlic clove, peeled and halved
1 tsp ground cumin
½ tsp crushed dried chilli flakes (optional)
2 tbsp extra-virgin olive oil
½ tsp flaked sea salt

1 Put all the ingredients in a food processor and season with lots of ground black pepper. Blitz until almost smooth. Adjust the seasoning to taste and blitz again but don't allow it to get too smooth.

2 Spoon into a bowl to serve.

COOK'S TIP

★ Keep covered in the fridge for up to 3 days or you can freeze for up to 1 month.

NON-FAST DAYS
Drizzle with olive oil and top with a sprinkling of toasted mixed seeds. Serve with fingers of toasted wholemeal pitta bread or wholemeal crispbread (see tip page 238).

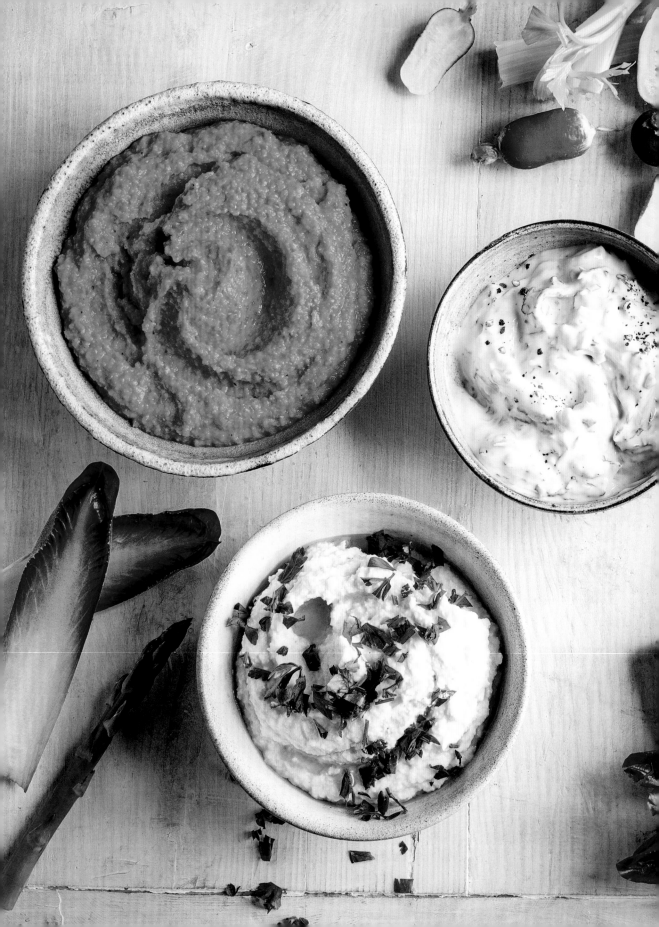

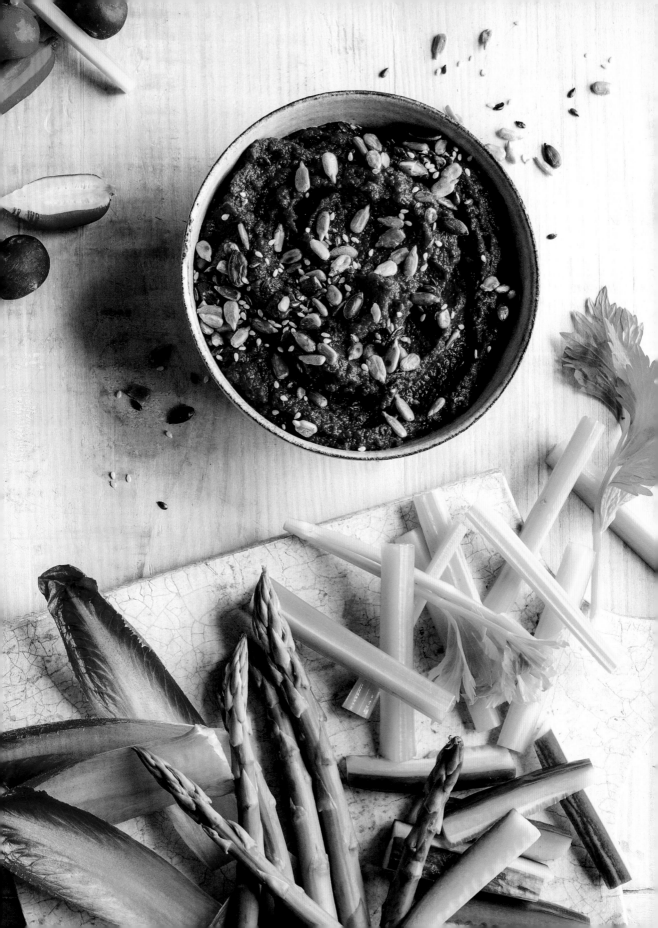

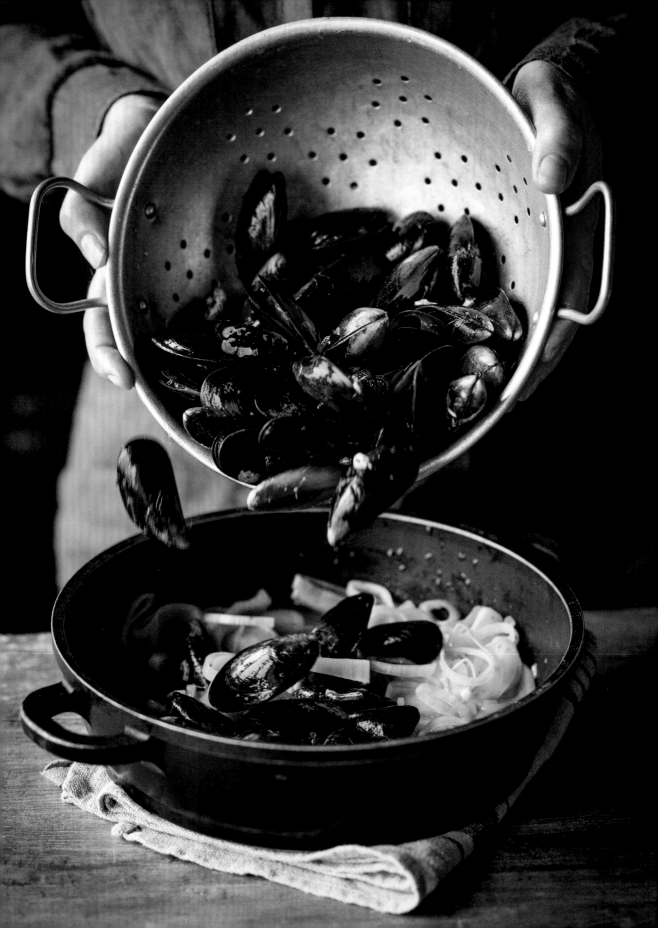

Fish and Shellfish

Fish and shellfish are among the healthiest foods on the planet. Eating fish, particularly oily fish that contains much-needed omega-3 oils such as salmon or mackerel, may reduce your risk of stroke or heart attack as well as reduce inflammation. And it is wonderfully quick and easy to prepare.

Michael's favourite seafood is mussels, which are also, happily, one of the most sustainable foods you can buy – so we have included his recipe for mussels in creamy tarragon sauce.

PER SERVING | **434cals** | PROTEIN **42g** | FAT **14g** | FIBRE **11g** | CARBS **29g**

Smoked haddock with lentils

SERVES 2

2 tbsp olive oil
½ medium onion, peeled
   and finely chopped
1 celery stick, trimmed
   and finely sliced
1 medium carrot, trimmed,
   halved lengthways and
   diagonally sliced
1 rosemary sprig or
   ¼ tsp dried rosemary
1 garlic clove, peeled and
   very finely sliced
1 × 250g sachet ready-cooked
   puy lentils
200ml vegetable stock
   (made with ½ stock cube)
2 × 140g smoked haddock
   or cod fillets, skinned
small handful roughly
   chopped fresh parsley
   leaves (optional)

NON-FAST DAYS
Top the fish with a poached egg
for an extra 78cals a serving, or
add 1–2 tablespoons of cooked
quinoa to the lentils just before
the end of the cooking time.
A splash of white wine is a
delicious addition to the stock.

A simple one-pan dish where the slightly smoky,
salty flavour of the fish holds its own and enhances
the earthiness of the lentils. Serve with a large
portion of cooked leafy greens.

1 Heat the oil in a non-stick frying pan or wide-based
saucepan over a low heat. Add the onion, celery and carrot
and gently fry for 5 minutes, or until soft but not browned.

2 Add the rosemary and garlic and cook for a few seconds
more, stirring. Tip the lentils into the pan and add the stock.
Bring to a gentle simmer then place the fish fillets on top.
Season well with ground black pepper and sprinkle with
chopped parsley, if using.

3 Cover the pan with a lid (or a heatproof plate) and cook
the fish for about 8 minutes, or until just beginning to flake
when prodded with a knife.

4 Divide the lentils between two warmed plates or bowls,
and top with the fish.

COOK'S TIPS

★ Buy your fish ready-skinned if you can, but if not,
place the fish on a board, skin-side down, and carefully
work a knife horizontally between the skin and the
fish using a gentle sawing motion until separated.
★ Use canned lentils if you can't find the sachets
in your local store.

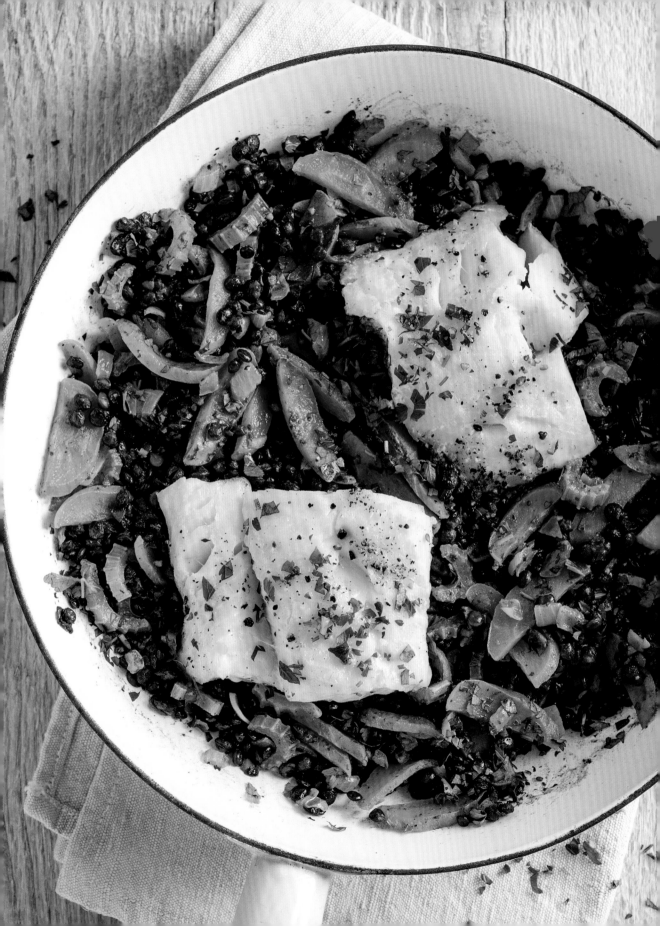

PER SERVING │ **368cals** │ PROTEIN **33g** │ FAT **26g** │ FIBRE **0.5g** │ CARBS **0.5g**

Pan-fried fish with lemon and parsley

SERVES 1

1 plaice fillet (around 175g), or other white fish fillet, thawed if frozen

15g butter

1 tbsp extra-virgin olive oil

1 tbsp fresh lemon juice

small bunch fresh parsley, leaves finely chopped (around 2 tbsp)

NON-FAST DAYS

Serve with a portion of warm white beans or some roasted vegetables. Add a knob of butter to your cooked greens or a generous splash of dressing to your salad. A serving of celeriac chips (see page 182) also goes well.

This is the ideal meal for one, but can be easily doubled up. Cook your vegetables, or prepare a salad, before you start frying the fish, as it takes less than 5 minutes. If you don't fancy plaice, sea bass or sea bream make good alternatives.

1 Season the fish on the skinless side with sea salt and black pepper.

2 Melt the butter with the oil in a large, non-stick frying pan over a medium heat. Add the plaice, skin-side down, and cook for 3 minutes. Carefully turn over and cook on the other side for a further 1–2 minutes, depending on the thickness of your fillet. (You can peel off the skin carefully at this point, if you like.)

3 Lift the plaice on to a warmed plate with a fish slice or spatula, turning on to the skin side. Return the pan to the heat, add the lemon juice and parsley and simmer for just a few seconds, stirring constantly.

4 Pour the buttery juices over the fish to serve.

COOK'S TIPS

★ Capers are delicious served with this fish. Simply add 1 tablespoon drained miniature capers at the same time as the lemon juice and parsley.

★ If you want the dish to be dairy free, omit the butter and reduce the calories by 28cals per serving.

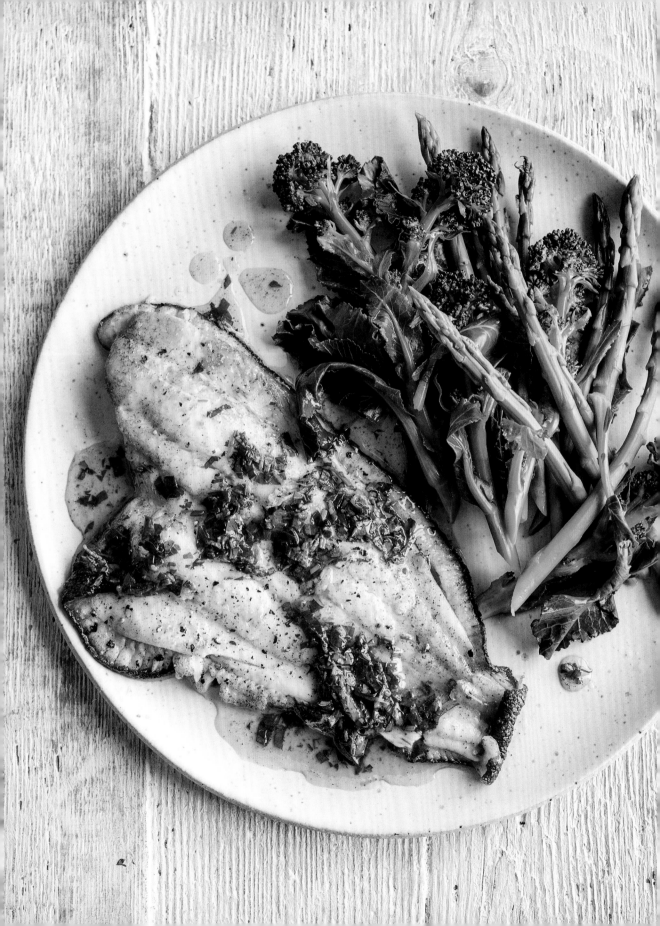

Crunchy fish bites

SERVES 2

1 medium egg
40g quick-cook polenta
    (fine cornmeal)
20g ground almonds
275g thick skinless white fish
    fillet (such as cod, haddock
    or pollock), cut into roughly
    3cm chunks
2 tbsp olive or rapeseed oil
lemon wedges, to serve

NON-FAST DAYS

Serve with good-quality, full-fat
mayonnaise mixed with a little
fresh lemon juice, or spoonfuls
of ready-made tartare sauce.
Or for a fish-and-chip-style meal,
serve with pea and broccoli mash
(see page 128) and celeriac
chips (see page 182).

Delicious chunky, white fish coated in a golden
covering made of polenta and ground almonds.
Once you have tasted these, you won't miss those
starchy, breaded or battered versions. Serve with
a large mixed salad, or freshly cooked greens.

1 Whisk the egg in a small bowl and season with sea salt
and black pepper. Combine the polenta and almonds in
a second bowl. Season with sea salt and black pepper.

2 One at a time, turn the pieces of fish in the beaten
egg until well covered, then toss in the polenta mixture.
Set aside on a plate.

3 Pour the oil into a large non-stick frying pan and place
over a medium heat. Fry the fish bites for 5–7 minutes,
depending on thickness, turning occasionally until
cooked through, golden brown and crisp on all sides.

4 Serve with lemon wedges for squeezing over.

COOK'S TIP

★ If you are cooking for one, freeze half the coated but
uncooked fish on a lined tray. Once solid, pop them into
a freezer container. You can fry them gently from frozen
– just add a few minutes to the cooking time.

Mediterranean fish bake

SERVES 2

1 medium red onion, peeled
    and cut into 12 wedges
1 red pepper, deseeded and cut
    into roughly 2cm chunks
1 medium courgette, trimmed,
    halved lengthways and
    cut into roughly 2cm slices
2 medium tomatoes, quartered
1½ tbsp olive oil
2 × 100g sea bass or
    sea bream fillets
40g pitted black olives
    (preferably Kalamata),
    drained
juice ½ large lemon,
    plus extra wedges to serve

NON-FAST DAYS

Roast small cubes of butternut
squash with the other vegetables
in the first step. Add a dressing
to the salad, if serving one
alongside, or drizzle the fish
with extra olive oil at the end.
A sprinkling of pine nuts
would also be lovely – add to
the baking tray for the last
2–3 minutes of cooking time.

Roasted Mediterranean-style vegetables work brilliantly with the fish in this simple traybake. Serve with a generous leafy green salad or a pile of thin green beans.

1 Preheat the oven to 200°C/fan 180°C/Gas 6.

2 Scatter the onion, pepper, courgette and tomato quarters over a large baking tray. Drizzle with 1 tablespoon of the oil and toss everything together. Season with sea salt and lots of ground black pepper and roast in the oven for 20 minutes.

3 Remove the tray from the oven and nestle the fish amongst the vegetables, skin-side down, and season with pepper. Scatter with the olives and squeeze the lemon juice over the top.

4 Return the tray to the oven for a further 8–10 minutes, or until the vegetables are tender and the fish is cooked through.

5 Divide the fish and vegetables between two warmed plates, drizzle with the remaining oil and serve with lemon wedges.

Swedish spicy carrot with cod

SERVES 2

2 large carrots (around 300g),
    trimmed and thickly sliced
1 garlic clove, peeled
15g fresh root ginger, peeled
15g butter
½ tbsp fresh lemon juice
2 × 150g thick, skinless cod
    fillets (or other white fish)
1 tbsp olive oil
good pinch crushed
    dried chilli flakes

NON-FAST DAYS
Scatter with a handful of toasted
almonds and drizzle with some
extra-virgin olive oil. Add a few
tablespoons of cooked puy
lentils to your plate.

Juicy cod steaks sitting on a creamy carrot purée.
Heaven. This recipe was inspired by a memorable
meal after a 5:2 conference in Stockholm. Serve
with half a plateful of cooked green vegetables, such
as long-stemmed broccoli, spring greens or kale.

1 Place the carrots, garlic and ginger in a medium
saucepan and cover with water. Bring to the boil then
reduce to a simmer and cook for 15 minutes or until soft.

2 Remove the pan from the heat, scoop out and reserve
a ladleful of water (around 100ml), then drain the carrot,
garlic and ginger. Return them to the pan with 3 tablespoons
of the reserved cooking water, the butter and lemon juice.
Using a stick blender, blitz the carrots to a soft, smooth
purée, adding a little extra cooking water if needed. Season
to taste with sea salt and ground black pepper. Set aside.

3 Season the cod fillets on all sides with sea salt and
black pepper. Heat the oil in a non-stick frying pan over
a medium heat. Add the cod and fry for 4 minutes. Turn
the fish, sprinkle with a few chilli flakes and cook on the
other side for a further 3–5 minutes, depending on the
thickness of each fillet. The cod is ready when it is just
beginning to flake into large chunks.

4 Spoon the purée on to two warmed plates and place
the fish on top.

COOK'S TIP

★ If you don't have a stick blender, use a food processor
or mash vigorously.

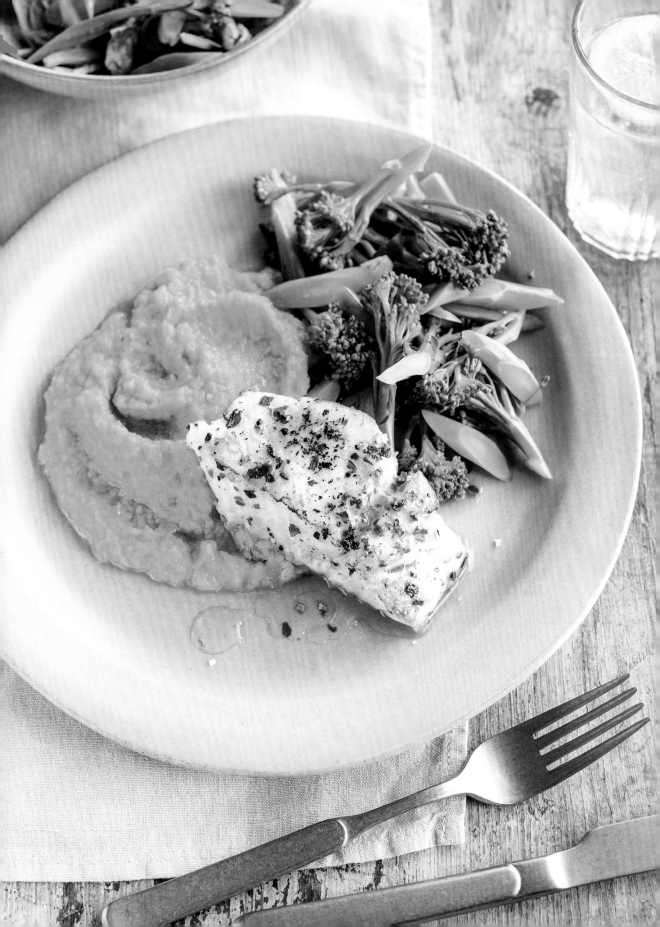

Ginger and chilli baked fish

SERVES 1

2 tsp olive or rapeseed oil

175g thick white fish fillet, such as cod (preferably skinned)

1 garlic clove, peeled and thinly sliced

15g stem ginger (around ½ ball), drained and cut into thin matchsticks

1 spring onion, trimmed and diagonally sliced

1 red bird's eye chilli, thinly sliced, or ¼ tsp crushed dried chilli flakes

juice ½ small lime, plus extra wedges to serve

handful fresh coriander leaves

NON-FAST DAYS

Serve with brown rice or a mixture of wild rice and brown basmati. Look out for pouches of ready-cooked rice in the supermarket for speed and convenience.

A super-easy baked fish dish which is perfect for one and can be easily multiplied for extra servings. We've used cod, but any thick white fish will work well. Serve with long-stemmed broccoli, mange tout or stir-fried vegetables to fill half the plate.

1 Preheat the oven to 200°C/fan 180°C/Gas 6. Place a rectangle of kitchen foil on a baking tray and drizzle with the oil.

2 Place the fish skin-side down on one half of the foil, leaving enough to cover. Sprinkle the fish with the garlic, ginger, spring onion and chilli, and squeeze over the lime juice. Season with sea salt and plenty of ground black pepper, then fold the foil over the fish to cover and roll up the edges to seal the fish inside. Don't make the parcel too tight as space is needed to create steam to cook the fish.

3 Bake in the oven for 12–15 minutes, or until the fish is cooked and flakes into large pieces when prodded with a fork.

4 Carefully open the foil parcel and lift the fish on to a warmed plate, using a fish slice or spatula. Spoon the cooking juices over the fish, top with lots of fresh coriander and serve with lime wedges.

COOK'S TIP

★ You'll usually find jars of stem ginger in syrup in the baking department of the supermarket, but 1 teaspoon freshly grated root ginger can be used instead.

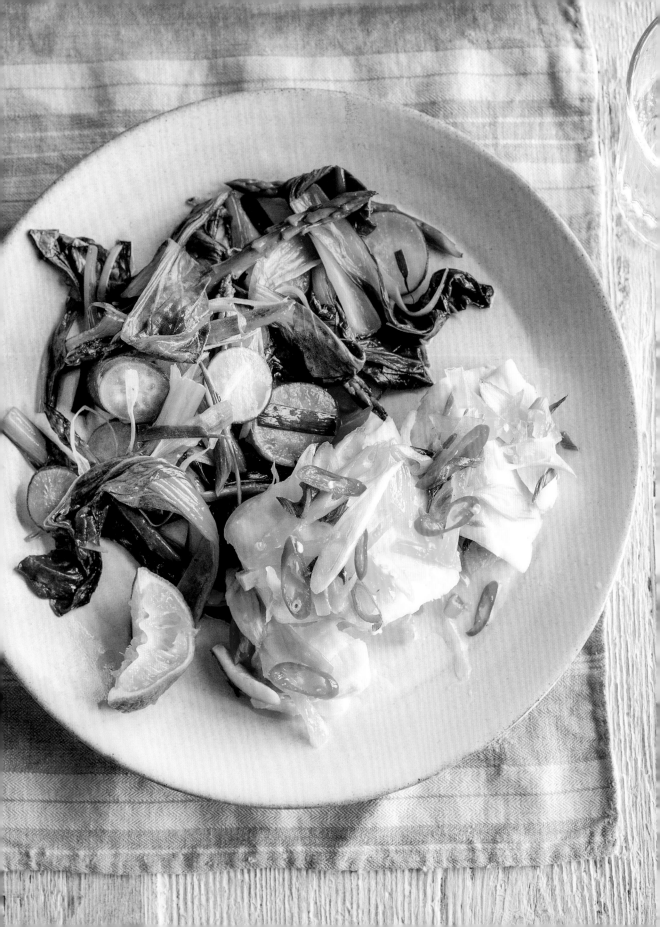

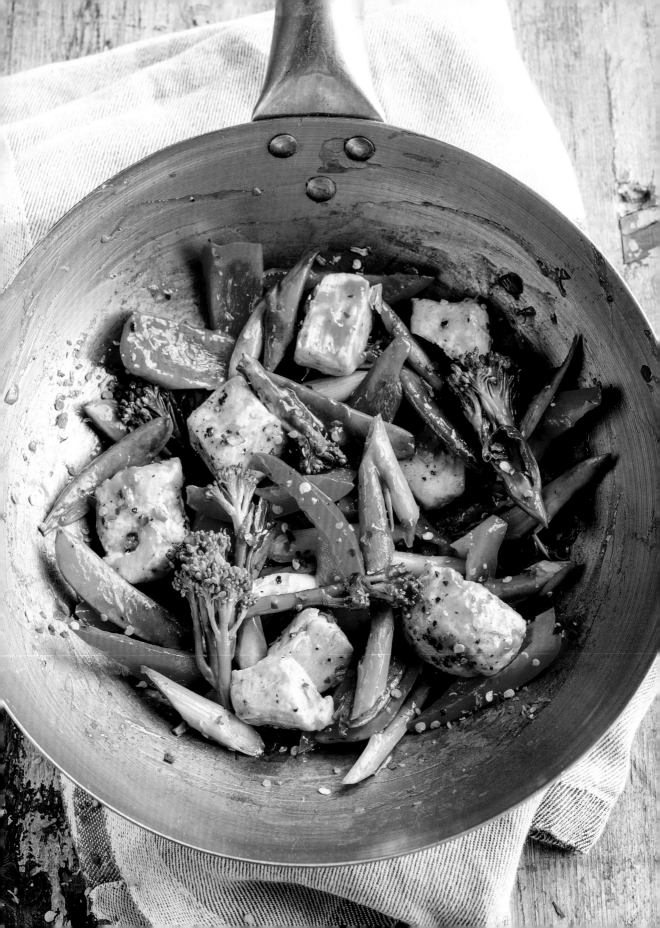

Stir-fry tuna with hoisin sauce

SERVES 1

1 × 110g fresh tuna steak, cut
 into roughly 3cm chunks
1 tbsp coconut or rapeseed oil
1 × 300–350g pack stir-fry
 vegetables
2 tbsp ready-made
 hoisin sauce
pinch crushed dried chilli
 flakes (optional)

NON-FAST DAYS
Serve with a small portion of
wholewheat noodles or brown
rice. You could also add a few
tablespoons of defrosted
edamame beans at stage 2.

This quick tuna dish is the perfect meal after a busy
day. Packs of ready-prepared stir-fry vegetables
save time and are easily available. Or make your
own combination with any fresh crispy vegetables.
And don't worry about the minor variations in the
calorie count of the stir-fried veg, just enjoy it!

1 Season the tuna on all sides with sea salt and ground
black pepper.

2 Heat the oil in a large non-stick frying pan or wok
over a high heat and stir-fry the tuna and vegetables
for 3–4 minutes, or according to the pack instructions,
and the tuna is lightly browned.

3 Drizzle over the hoisin sauce and toss with the fish
and vegetables for 20–30 seconds more.

4 Sprinkle with the chilli flakes, if using, and serve
immediately.

COOK'S TIP

★ Use any firm fish you like for this easy dish; salmon
and cod work well. Prawns can be used, as can thin
strips of chicken breast. You'll need to adjust the calories
if you make any substitutions – the tuna is 118cals.

PER SERVING | **507cals** | PROTEIN **34.5g** | FAT **39.5g** | FIBRE **2g** | CARBS **2.5g**

Leek and salmon quiche in a dish

SERVES 2

1 tbsp olive oil, plus
    extra for greasing
1 medium leek, trimmed
    and thinly sliced (around
    100g prepared weight)
1 garlic clove, peeled
    and crushed
generous handful young
    spinach leaves (around 50g)
100g cooked salmon
    fillet, skinned
4 large eggs
½ tbsp fresh thyme leaves
    or ½ tsp dried thyme
45g full-fat crème fraîche
15g Parmesan, medium grated

NON-FAST DAYS
Add a dressing to the salad,
if serving one alongside, a bit
of butter on the veg and include
a few tablespoons of cooked
pearl barley or lentils.

Abandoning the pastry crust makes this easy salmon quiche much lower in calories and carbs. Enjoy it warm with a large green and red leaf salad or cold as a nutritious, high-protein addition to a packed lunch.

1 Preheat the oven to 190°C/fan 170°C/Gas 5. Generously oil a small ovenproof baking dish, to hold around 900ml of liquid, or two small dishes.

2 Heat the oil in a medium non-stick frying pan over a medium heat. Add the leek and gently fry for 3 minutes, or until softened but not browned, stirring.

3 Add the garlic and spinach, a handful at a time, and cook for about 2 minutes or until the spinach has wilted and softened, stirring constantly. Transfer to a sieve and press out the excess liquid from the spinach with the back of a spoon. Tip the leeks and spinach into the oiled dish or divide between the dishes.

4 Flake the salmon into chunky pieces and add to the leeks and spinach, spreading loosely over the base of the dish.

5 Whisk the eggs, thyme and crème fraîche in a small bowl. Add 2 tablespoons of the Parmesan, season with salt and lots of ground black pepper and stir well.

6 Pour the egg mixture gently over the salmon and veg. Sprinkle with the remaining Parmesan and bake for about 25 minutes (15–20 minutes if using two dishes), or until slightly puffed up, golden brown and just set.

COOK'S TIP

★ Use freshly snipped dill or chopped parsley instead of the thyme, if you like.

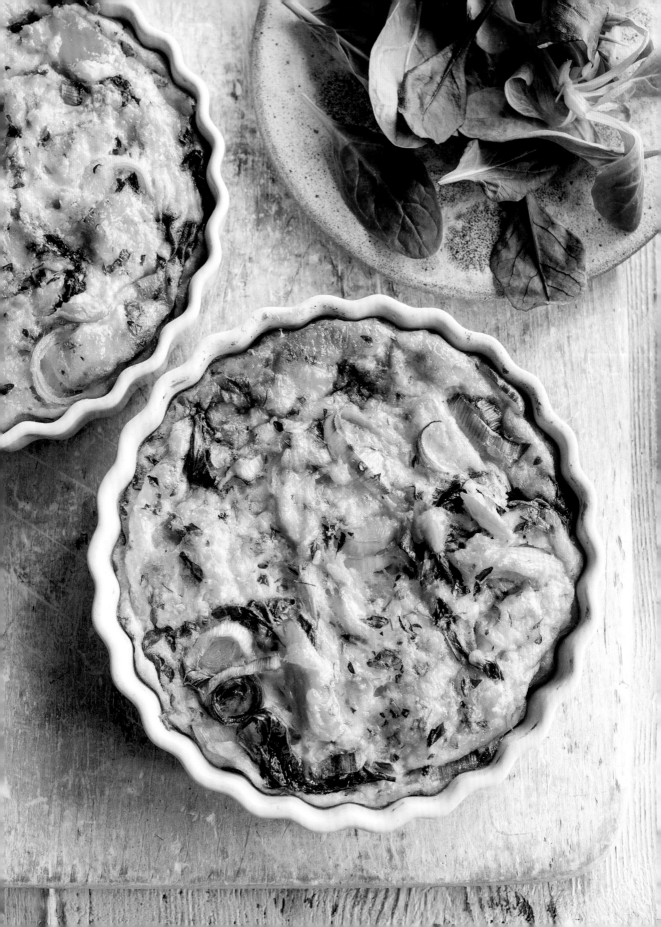

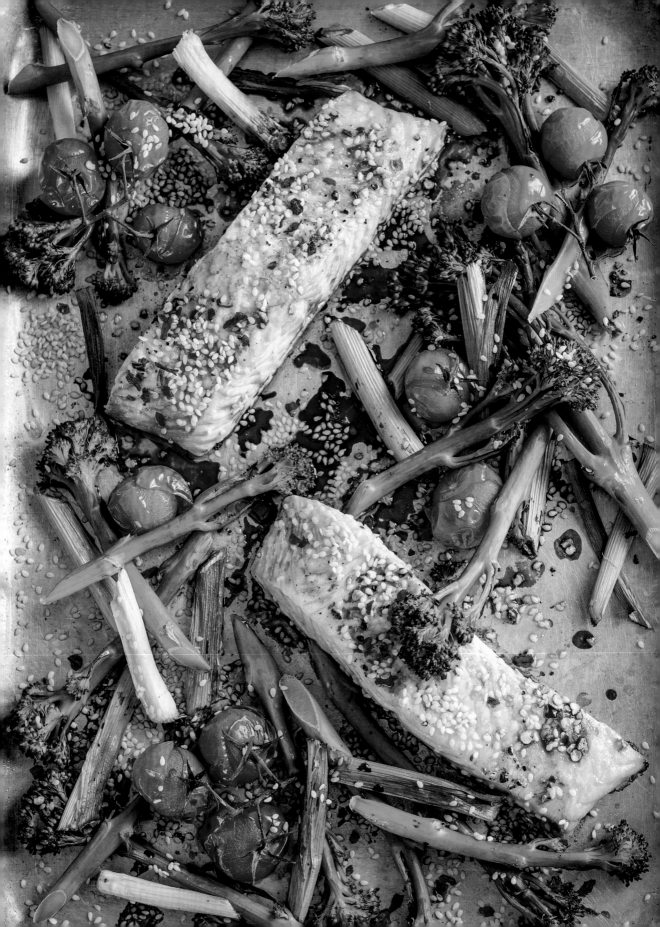

Sesame salmon with broccoli and tomatoes

SERVES 2

2 tsp olive or rapeseed oil
2 × 125g salmon fillets
6 spring onions, trimmed
    and each cut into 3 pieces
12 cherry tomatoes
200g long-stemmed
    broccoli, trimmed
1 tbsp dark soy sauce
1 tsp sesame oil
½ tsp crushed dried
    chilli flakes
1 tsp sesame seeds

NON-FAST DAYS
Serve with wholegrain noodles
or brown rice. Or try pea, bean
or lentil pasta for a delicious
and gluten-free alternative.
Soba noodles work well, too.

This is wonderful served hot for supper or cold for
lunch on the go. If you don't fancy salmon, any other
chunky fish fillet will work well.

1 Preheat the oven to 200°C/fan 180°C/Gas 6. Drizzle
a baking tray with the oil.

2 Place the salmon fillets in the tray, skin-side down,
add the spring onions and tomatoes and season with
lots of ground black pepper. Bake for 8 minutes.

3 Meanwhile, third fill a pan with water and bring to
the boil. Add the broccoli and return to the boil. Cook
for 4 minutes then drain.

4 Remove the tray from the oven and add the broccoli.
Drizzle the soy sauce and sesame oil over the fish.
Sprinkle everything with the chilli flakes and sesame
seeds and return to the oven for a further 3–4 minutes,
or until the salmon is just cooked.

5 Divide between two warmed plates and serve.

COOK'S TIP

★ You can test the salmon is ready by prodding with
the side of a fork. It should flake into large pieces and
look pale pink and opaque on the outside but slightly
translucent right in the middle.

Baked salmon with pea and broccoli mash

SERVES 2

15g butter, plus extra
  for greasing
2 × 125g fresh salmon fillets
150g frozen peas
150g broccoli, cut into small
  florets and stalks thinly
  sliced
1 tbsp finely chopped fresh
  mint (optional)
lemon wedges, to serve

NON-FAST DAYS
Toss cubes of peeled butternut
squash in olive oil and roast on a
baking tray for 15 minutes before
placing the tray with the fish on
the rack above. Cook both trays
for a further 10–12 minutes.

This is easy-peasy, ready in less than 15 minutes.

1 Preheat the oven to 200°C/fan 180°C/Gas 6.
Line a small baking tray with foil and grease lightly
with butter.

2 Place the salmon on the foil, skin-side down, and
season with a little salt and lots of ground black pepper.
Bake for 10–12 minutes, depending on thickness.

3 Meanwhile, to make the pea and broccoli mash, half
fill a pan with water and bring to the boil. Add the peas
and broccoli and return to the boil. Cook for 5 minutes,
or until the broccoli is tender. Reserve a small ladleful
of the cooking water (around 75ml), then drain the
vegetables and return them to the pan.

4 Add the butter, mint, if using, and 3 tablespoons
of the reserved cooking water to the pan and blitz with
a stick blender until almost smooth. Season to taste,
adding a little extra water to loosen, if needed.

5 Divide the mash between two warmed plates and
top with the roasted salmon; it should lift off the foil,
leaving the skin behind. Serve with lemon wedges.

COOK'S TIP

★ If you don't have a stick blender, blitz the peas and
broccoli in a food processor then return to the pan.
Or simply mash vigorously.

Prawn nasi goreng

SERVES 2

2 tbsp coconut or rapeseed oil

1 medium onion,
    peeled and diced

1 red pepper, deseeded and
    cut into roughly 2cm chunks

½ small Savoy cabbage, leaves
    thinly sliced (about 275g
    prepared weight)

2 garlic cloves, peeled
    and thinly sliced

20g fresh root ginger,
    peeled and finely grated

½–1 tsp crushed dried
    chilli flakes (to taste)

200g cauliflower rice (see tip)

2 tbsp dark soy sauce

150g cooked, peeled prawns,
    thawed if frozen

generous handful fresh
    coriander, leaves roughly
    chopped (optional)

20g roasted peanuts,
    roughly chopped

NON-FAST DAYS
Swap the cauliflower rice
for cooked brown rice.

My mother used to make a wonderful wok-ful of nasi goreng, garnished with fresh prawns and crispy onions. This is a quick, low-carb version that uses cauliflower 'rice' instead of basmati. Have everything ready before you start to cook as it will only take a few minutes.

1 Heat the oil in a large non-stick frying pan or wok over a medium–hot setting. Stir-fry the onion, red pepper and cabbage for 2–3 minutes, stirring frequently.

2 Add the garlic, ginger, chilli and cauliflower rice and stir-fry for 2–3 minutes more, or until the cauliflower is hot.

3 Add the soy sauce, prawns and half the coriander, if using, and cook for a further 1–2 minutes, stirring and tossing until the prawns are hot. Add more soy sauce to taste.

4 Divide between two bowls and top with the chopped nuts and the remaining coriander, if using. Add some more chilli flakes, if you like it hot.

COOK'S TIPS

★ For extra protein, top with 2 medium eggs, fried in 1 teaspoon of oil. This will add an extra 94cals per serving.
★ To make the cauliflower rice: Hold a small cauliflower at the stalk end and coarsely grate in short, sharp movements in a downward direction only to create tiny shavings of cauliflower resembling grains of rice. You can also do this in a food processor but don't let the pieces get too small or they will turn to a paste. If it makes life easier, you can buy ready-made cauliflower rice.
★ For a vegetarian version, swap the prawns (52cals per serving) for 100g tofu fried in 2 tablespoons of oil (143cals per serving).

Thai curry with prawns

SERVES 2

1 tbsp coconut or rapeseed oil
1 red pepper, deseeded and cut
    into roughly 2cm chunks
4 spring onions, trimmed
    and thickly sliced
20g fresh root ginger,
    peeled and finely grated
3 tbsp Thai red or
    green curry paste
½ × 400ml can coconut milk
100g mange tout or
    sugar-snap peas, halved
1 red chilli, finely sliced,
    or ½ tsp crushed dried
    chilli flakes (optional)
200g large cooked peeled
    prawns, thawed if frozen

NON-FAST DAYS
Serve with brown rice
or wholewheat noodles.

A creamy curry, full of Thai flavours and remarkably
filling. Super-quick and easy, too.

1 Heat the oil in a large non-stick frying pan or wok over
a medium–high heat and stir-fry the pepper for 2 minutes.
Add the spring onions, ginger and curry paste and cook
for 1 minute more, stirring.

2 Pour the coconut milk into the pan and bring to
a gentle simmer.

3 Add the mange tout or sugar snap peas and chilli,
if using. Return to a simmer and cook for 2 minutes,
stirring regularly.

4 Add the prawns and heat for 1–2 minutes, or until hot.
Adding a splash of water if the sauce thickens too much.

5 Serve with freshly cooked cauliflower rice (see page 242).

COOK'S TIPS

★ Thai pastes do vary, so try and pick a good-quality
one for the best depth of flavour.
★ For half a can of coconut milk, tip the contents of a
400ml can into a measuring jug and whisk until as smooth
as possible. Pour 200ml of the liquid into a bowl, cover
and keep for another recipe. Use within 2 days, or pour
into a lidded container and freeze for up to 1 month.

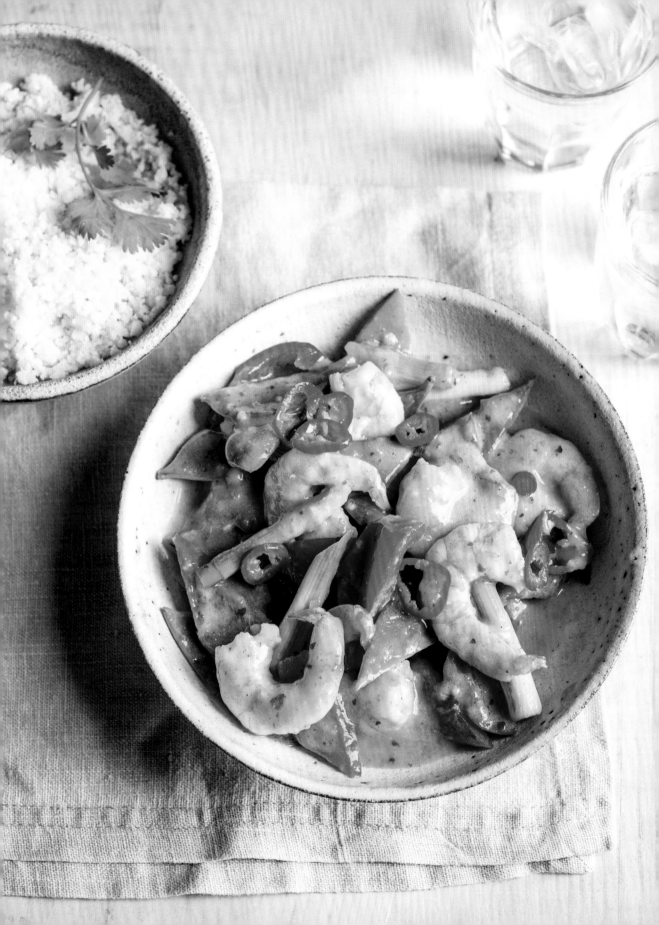

Mussels with creamy tarragon sauce

SERVES 2

1kg fresh, live mussels

1 tbsp olive oil

1 medium leek, trimmed
    and thinly sliced (around
    100g prepared weight)

2 garlic cloves, peeled
    and thinly sliced

100ml dry white wine

75g full-fat crème fraîche

3–4 fresh tarragon stalks
    (around 5g), leaves picked
    and roughly chopped,
    or 1 tsp dried tarragon

NON-FAST DAYS
Serve with celeriac chips
(see page 182).

Mussels make a fabulous, cheap, low-calorie yet high-protein meal. If you haven't cooked them before, don't be put off, they are incredibly easy and the quality of farmed mussels in the UK is superb. Serve with a 50g slice of brown sourdough or wholegrain bread (119cals).

1 Tip the mussels into the sink, scrub well under cold running water and remove the 'beards'. Discard any mussels with damaged shells or those that don't close immediately when tapped on the side of the sink. Put the good ones into a colander.

2 Heat the oil in a deep, lidded, wide-based saucepan or shallow casserole, over a low heat. Add the leek and garlic and very gently fry for 2–3 minutes, or until softened but not browned.

3 Add the white wine, crème fraîche and tarragon and season generously. Increase the heat under the pan and bring the wine to a simmer.

4 Stir in the mussels, cover tightly with a lid and cook for about 4 minutes, or until most of the mussels have steamed open. Stir well, then cover and cook for a further 1–2 minutes or until the rest are cooked.

5 Divide the mussels between two bowls, removing any that haven't opened, and pour the tarragon broth over the top.

COOK'S TIP

★ If you can't get hold of tarragon, use freshly chopped parsley or dill instead.

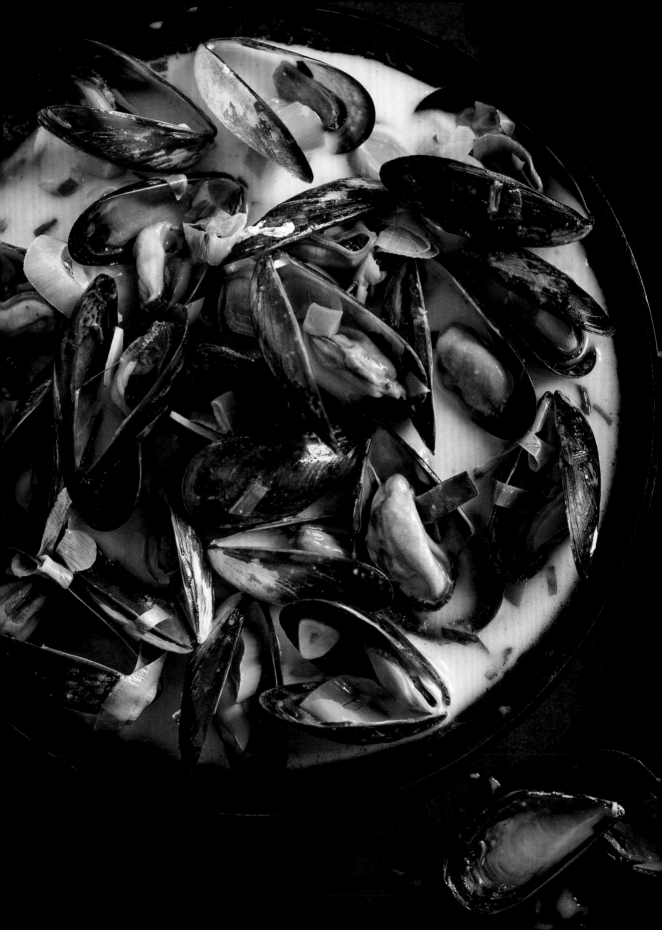

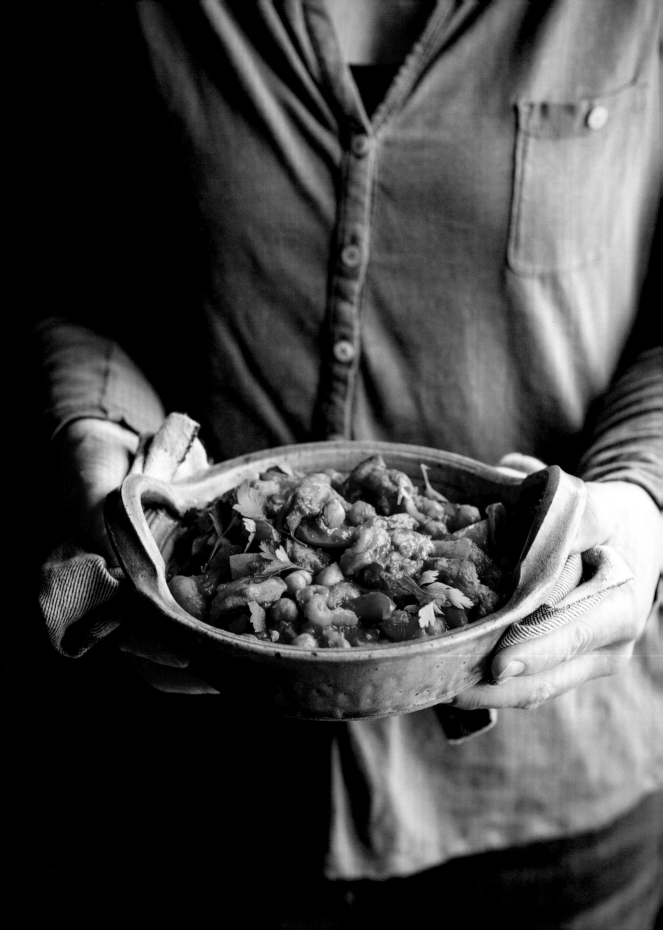

Chicken
and Turkey

Chicken and turkey are high-quality sources of protein, particularly when you are fasting. In this chapter, we have included lower-carb versions of classic dishes, such as Chicken goujons with Parmesan crumb, and a variety of curries, casseroles and bakes. Aim to look for responsibly sourced options.

PER SERVING | **385cals** | PROTEIN **58g** | FAT **17g** | FIBRE **0g** | CARBS **0g**

Roast chicken thighs with lemon

SERVES 2

4 bone-in chicken thighs
    (each around 150g)
1–2 lemons, juice of 1
    (around 2 tbsp), the other
    quartered (optional)
1 tbsp olive oil
2 tbsp fresh thyme leaves or
    2–3 sprigs fresh rosemary,
    roughly chopped (or use
    1 tsp dried herbs)
1 bulb garlic, halved (optional)

NON-FAST DAYS
Serve with roasted butternut
squash and/or 3 tablespoons
of cooked quinoa or brown
or wild rice.

This juicy, herb-infused chicken is perfect served
with a large green and coloured leaf salad, dressed
with our Simple salad dressing (see page 241), or
a generous serving of freshly cooked vegetables.
It works brilliantly on the barbecue, too.

1 If cooking the chicken straight away, preheat the oven
to 200°C/fan 180°C/Gas 6.

2 Put the chicken in a bowl with the lemon juice and oil.
Add the thyme or rosemary and season with sea salt and
lots of ground black pepper. Toss well together. If you have
time, cover and leave to marinate in the fridge for at least
1 hour and up to 4 hours.

3 Place the chicken, skin-side up, in a roasting tin with
the herbs and quartered lemon, if using, and bake for
15 minutes. Remove the tin from the oven, add the garlic,
if using, and cook for a further 20–25 minutes, or until
the chicken is lightly browned, tender and cooked all
the way through.

COOK'S TIPS

★ If you remove the skin before eating, you will save
25cals per serving.
★ Add extra herbs for garnish about 10 minutes before
the end of the cooking time, if you like.

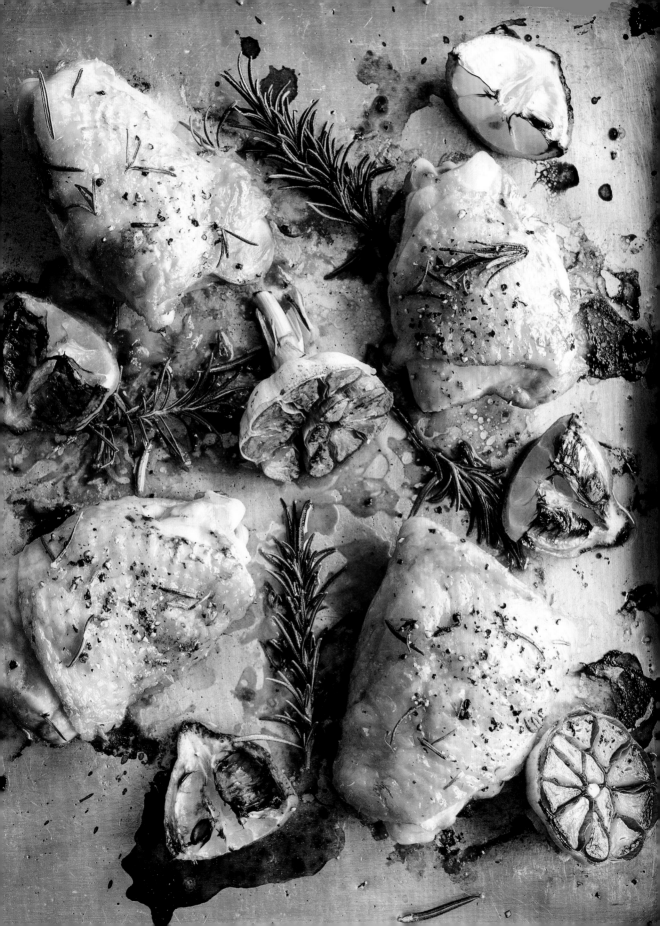

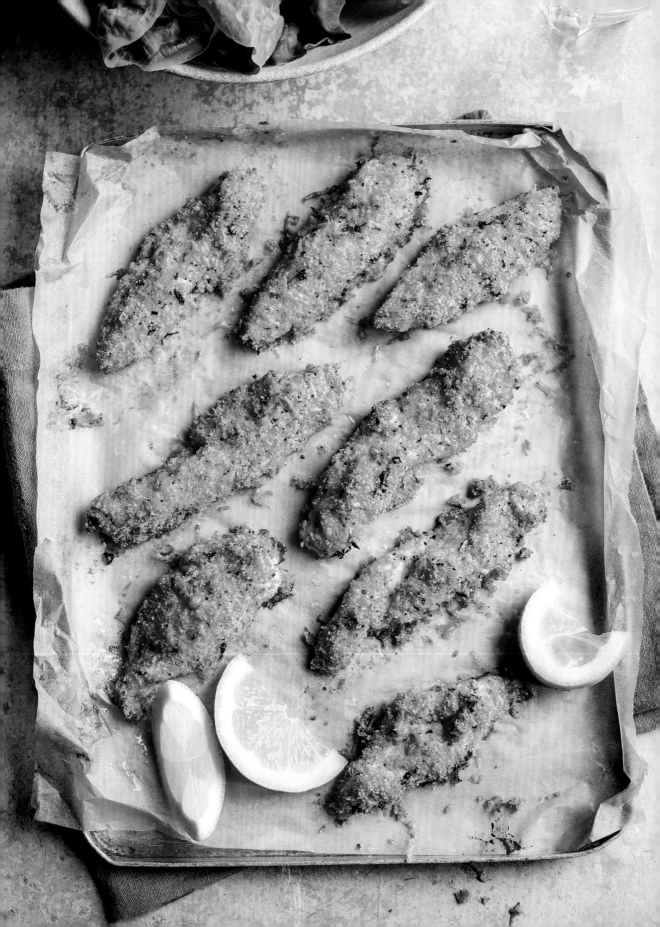

Chicken goujons with Parmesan crumb

SERVES 2
1 medium egg
50g Parmesan, finely grated
25g quick-cook polenta
    (fine cornmeal)
½ tsp dried thyme
½ tsp paprika (not smoked)
2 boneless, skinless chicken
    breast fillets (around 400g),
    each cut into 4–5 thin strips
lemon wedges, to serve

NON-FAST DAYS
Serve with a lemon mayo by
combining a good-quality, full-fat
mayonnaise with a little grated
lemon zest and juice. You could
also serve with a portion of
celeriac chips (see page 182)
and a pile of cooked petits pois.

Tender chicken breast pieces with a crunchy golden
Parmesan coating. Delicious served warm with a large
mixed salad, dressed with our Simple salad dressing
(see page 241), or with steamed sliced courgettes
or a generous portion of mange tout.

1 Preheat the oven to 200°C/fan 180°C/Gas 6. Line
a large baking tray with non-stick baking paper.

2 Whisk the egg in a medium bowl until smooth. Combine
the Parmesan, polenta, thyme and paprika with some fine
sea salt and a good grinding of black pepper in a separate
bowl. Scatter half the mixture over a large plate.

3 Dip the chicken strips, one at a time, into the egg then
coat in the Parmesan crumb. Top up the crumbs on the
plate when the first batch is used up.

4 Place the goujons on the baking tray and bake
for 12–14 minutes, or until crisp, golden brown and
cooked through.

5 Divide between two plates and serve with a squeeze
of lemon.

COOK'S TIP

★ You can buy chicken mini fillets in packs from most
supermarkets, which would make the prep quicker.

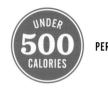
One-pot roast chicken

SERVES 4

2 rashers smoked back bacon,
    cut into roughly 2cm strips
1 medium onion,
    peeled and sliced
1 medium chicken
    (around 1.6kg)
1 tbsp olive oil
150g baby carrots, trimmed
150g baby parsnips,
    peeled and trimmed
200ml hot chicken stock
    (made with 1 stock cube)
100ml dry white wine,
    or extra stock
1 tbsp fresh thyme
    leaves or ½ tsp dried
    thyme (optional)
200g frozen peas

NON-FAST DAYS
Increase your portion size.

An all-in-one chicken dish, which is perfect for
a family lunch.

1 Preheat the oven to 200°C/fan 180°C/Gas 6.

2 Combine the bacon and onion in a medium flame-proof
casserole and place the chicken on top. Drizzle with the oil
and season with sea salt and ground black pepper. Roast for
30 minutes uncovered, until the chicken is golden brown.

3 Remove from the oven, transfer the chicken to a plate
and add the carrots and parsnips to the casserole. Pour
in the stock and wine, if using, and scatter with the
thyme, if using. Place the chicken on top of the vegetables,
cover the casserole with a lid and bake for a further
45–55 minutes or until the vegetables are tender and
the chicken is cooked through.

4 Lift the chicken carefully out on to a warmed platter.
Place the casserole on the hob and skim off any fat that
has risen to the surface. Stir in the peas and bring the
liquid to a boil (take care as the pan will be very hot).
Boil hard for 2–3 minutes, or until the pan juices are
reduced by half. Season to taste.

5 Carve the chicken into chunky pieces and serve in
deep plates or bowls with the vegetables and cooking
liquor poured over.

COOK'S TIP

★ Your casserole needs to be large enough to hold the
chicken with the lid on. If you don't have one to hand,
cook the chicken and vegetables in a sturdy roasting
tin and cover tightly with foil instead of a lid.

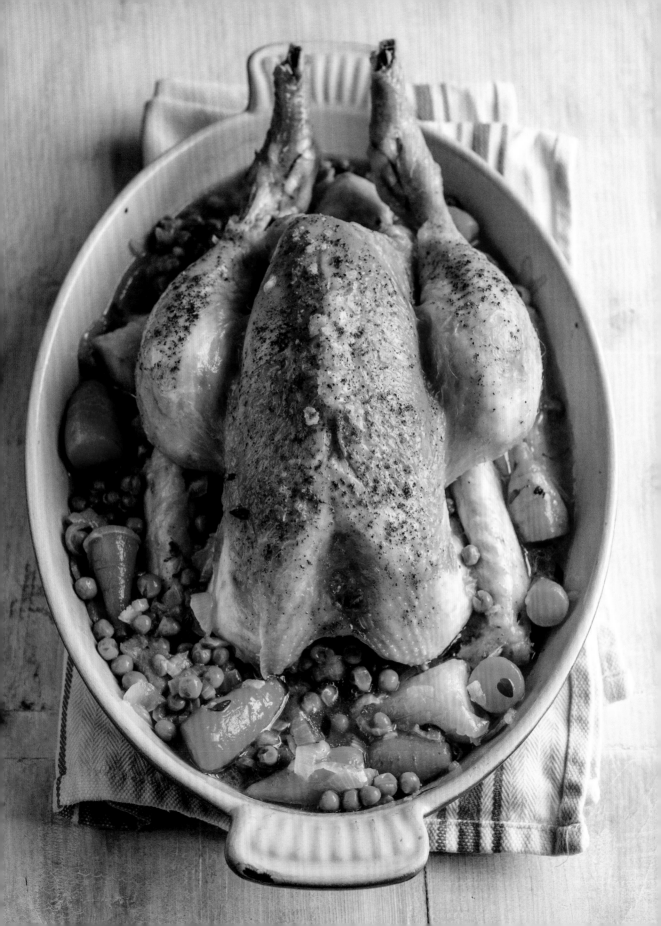

Simple chicken casserole

SERVES 4

2 tbsp olive oil

6 boneless, skinless
chicken thighs
(around 600g), quartered

2 smoked back bacon rashers,
cut into roughly 2cm strips

1 large onion, peeled
and finely sliced

150g button mushrooms,
halved or sliced if large

1 × 400g can chopped tomatoes

3 medium carrots, trimmed
and cut into roughly
1cm slices

1 chicken stock cube

1 tsp mixed dried herbs

NON-FAST DAYS
Increase the portion size and
serve with 2–3 tablespoons
of cooked brown rice or quinoa.
You can also add a can of
cannellini or butterbeans to
the casserole, along with an
extra drizzle of olive oil.

Tasty comfort food suitable for a family supper that
can also be reheated the next day, or frozen for another
time. Serve with lots of freshly cooked green vegetables,
such as cabbage, broccoli, green beans or kale.

1 Preheat the oven to 200°C/fan 180°C/Gas 6.

2 Heat the oil in a flame-proof casserole dish over a medium
heat. Add the chicken, bacon, onion and mushrooms,
season with a little sea salt and lots of ground black pepper
and cook for 6–8 minutes, stirring regularly until the chicken
is coloured on all sides and the onion is lightly browned.

3 Add the tomatoes, carrots, crumbled stock cube and
dried herbs. Pour over 400ml cold water and stir well.
Bring to a simmer then cover with a lid and cook in the
oven for 40 minutes, or until the chicken is tender.

UNDER **400** CALORIES

Chicken wrapped in Parma ham

SERVES 4

4 boneless, skinless chicken
    breasts (each around 150g)
4 slices Parma ham
    or prosciutto
2 tbsp olive oil
1 medium onion, peeled
    and finely chopped
2 garlic cloves, peeled
    and crushed
1 × 400g can chopped tomatoes
    or 500g passata
1 tsp dried oregano
200g young spinach leaves
25g Parmesan, finely grated

NON-FAST DAYS
Serve the salad with an olive
oil dressing.

A very popular dish in our house. Serve with
a large mixed salad.

1 Place the chicken on a board and cover with a sheet of
cling film. Bash with a rolling pin to flatten until around
2cm thick. Season with sea salt and ground black pepper
and wrap each of the breasts in a slice of Parma ham.

2 Heat 1 tablespoon of the oil in a large, non-stick frying
pan or shallow flame-proof casserole dish. Add the
wrapped chicken and fry on each side over a medium
heat for 3–4 minutes, or until lightly browned. Transfer
to a plate.

3 Add the remaining oil to the pan with the onion and
gently fry for 5 minutes, then stir in the garlic and cook
for a few seconds more.

4 Add the chopped tomatoes or passata, oregano, 300ml
water and the spinach, a handful at a time (the pan will
look very full). Bring to a gentle simmer and cook for
2–3 minutes, or until the spinach is very soft, stirring
occasionally. Season the sauce.

5 Return the chicken to the pan and nestle into the sauce.
Simmer gently for 18–20 minutes, or until the chicken
is tender and thoroughly cooked, adding an extra splash
of water if needed. Sprinkle with Parmesan to serve.

COOK'S TIP

★ Freeze any leftover breasts with the sauce in lidded
containers for up to 1 month. Defrost thoroughly, then
reheat in a microwave or slice the chicken and reheat with
the sauce in a frying pan until piping hot throughout.

Easy chicken tagine

SERVES 2

2 tbsp olive oil

1 medium onion, peeled
    and thinly sliced

3 boneless, skinless
    chicken thighs
    (around 300g), quartered

1½ tsp ground cumin

1½ tsp ground coriander

¼ tsp ground cinnamon

1 red pepper, deseeded and
    cut into roughly 3cm chunks

1 × 400g can chopped tomatoes

1 × 210g can chickpeas,
    drained (around 130g
    drained weight)

4 dried apricots (around 25g),
    roughly chopped

1 chicken stock cube

handful fresh coriander or
    parsley, leaves roughly
    chopped, to serve

NON-FAST DAYS
Increase the portion size
and serve with 3 tablespoons
of quinoa or bulgur wheat.

A filling Moroccan-inspired casserole with lovely
fibre-rich chickpeas. Don't be put off by the number
of ingredients – once the chicken is browned it's an
easy throw-it-in-the-oven number. Serve with a large
portion of green beans or a generous leafy salad.

1 Preheat the oven to 200°C/fan 180°C/Gas 6.

2 Heat the oil in a medium flame-proof casserole over
a medium heat. Add the onion and chicken and gently
fry for 6–8 minutes, or until the onion is lightly browned,
stirring regularly.

3 Sprinkle with the spices and cook for a few seconds
more, stirring.

4 Add the pepper, tomatoes, chickpeas, apricots and
crumbled stock cube. Pour in 250ml water, season with
sea salt and plenty of ground black pepper and bring
to a simmer. Cover with a lid and cook in the oven for
45 minutes, or until the chicken is tender and the
sauce has thickened.

5 Sprinkle with coriander or parsley to serve.

COOK'S TIP

★ For a more fiery taste, add 1 tablespoon harissa paste
with the tomatoes. For a meat-free version, omit the
chicken, which is 163cals per serving, use a veggie stock
cube and add 200g cubed butternut squash instead.

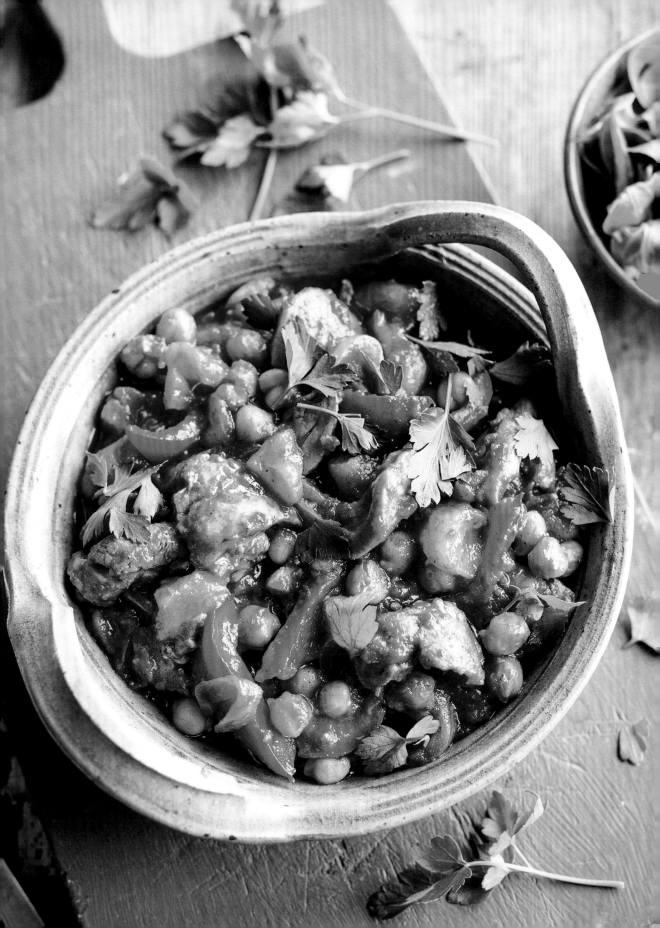

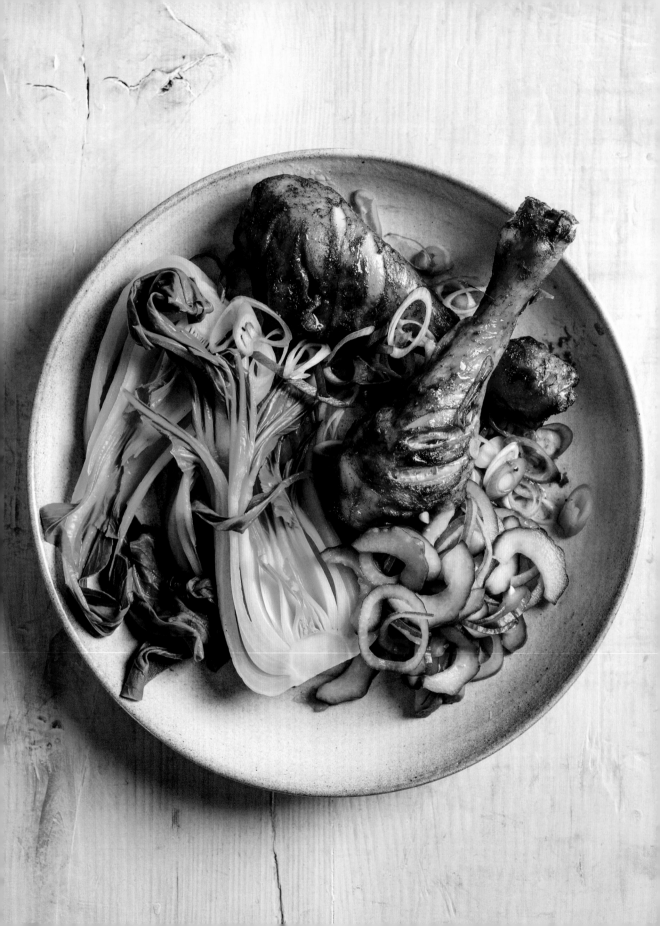

Chinese-style drumsticks

SERVES 4

2 tsp Chinese five spice powder

4 tbsp dark soy sauce

2 tsp sesame oil

2 garlic cloves, peeled and
crushed

8 chicken drumsticks

2 spring onions, trimmed and
finely sliced (optional)

NON-FAST DAYS
Enjoy with 3 tablespoons
of brown rice or quinoa.

These can be oven-baked but are great for cooking
on the barbecue, too. Serve with steamed pak choi
or spring greens, or a large mixed salad.

1 Put the five spice, soy sauce, sesame oil and garlic
in a large bowl and mix thoroughly. Slash each chicken
drumstick through the thickest part 2–3 times and add
to the marinade. Mix well. Cover and leave in the fridge
to marinate for at least 30 minutes, or ideally several
hours, turning occasionally.

2 Preheat the oven to 220°C/fan 200°C/Gas 7. Line
a large baking tray with foil.

3 Place the drumsticks on the prepared tray, reserving
any marinade left in the bowl, and bake for 20 minutes.

4 Remove from the oven, brush the chicken generously
with the remaining marinade and return to the oven for
a further 10–15 minutes, or until the chicken is tender
and cooked throughout.

5 Garnish with the spring onions, if using, to serve.

COOK'S TIP

★ Make quick pickled cucumber to serve with the
drumsticks by mixing half a very thinly sliced small red
onion with half a deseeded and thinly sliced cucumber.
Top with 1½ tablespoons live cider vinegar and season
with a generous pinch of sea salt. Leave to stand for
30 minutes.

| PER SERVING | **427cals** | PROTEIN **46g** | FAT **21g** | FIBRE **4g** | CARBS **11.5g**

Chicken tikka masala

SERVES 2

1 tbsp tikka curry paste

4 tbsp full-fat live
   Greek yoghurt

2 boneless, skinless chicken
   breasts (around 350g), cut
   into roughly 3cm chunks

1 tbsp coconut or rapeseed oil

fresh coriander, to serve
   (optional)

½ red chilli, sliced, to serve
   (optional)

For the masala sauce

1 tbsp coconut or rapeseed oil

1 medium onion, peeled and
   finely chopped

2 garlic cloves, peeled
   and crushed

15g fresh root ginger,
   peeled and finely grated

2 tbsp tikka curry paste

1 tbsp tomato purée

NON-FAST DAYS

Serve with a portion of Minty
yoghurt raitha (see page 106)
and 2–3 heaped tablespoons of
brown rice or a wholemeal roti.

A healthy version of a favourite curry, which is much
better than a take-away. Choose a good-quality tikka
curry paste. Serve with steamed greens or cauliflower
rice (see page 242).

1 Combine the curry paste, yoghurt and 2 generous
pinches of sea salt in a bowl. Add the chicken and mix
until well coated. Cover and leave to marinate in the fridge
for at least 1 hour, preferably longer or even overnight.

2 Fifteen minutes before you are ready to serve, make
the sauce. Heat the oil in a large non-stick saucepan over
a medium heat. Add the onion and fry gently for 5 minutes,
or until softened, then stir in the garlic, ginger and curry
paste and cook for 1½ minutes more. Pour 300ml water
into the pan, stir in the tomato purée and bring to a simmer.
Cook for 5 minutes, then remove the pan from the heat
and use a hand blender to blitz the sauce. Set aside.

3 Heat the remaining oil in a large non-stick frying pan
over a medium–high heat and fry the marinated chicken
for 3 minutes, or until lightly browned, turning regularly.

4 Add the prepared sauce to the pan and bring to a simmer.
Cook for 3–4 minutes, or until the chicken is thoroughly
cooked, stirring constantly. Add a splash of water if the
sauce thickens too much.

5 Sprinkle with the chopped coriander and chilli, if using,
to serve.

COOK'S TIP

★ If you don't have a stick blender, you can leave out the
blitzing but the sauce won't be as smooth and creamy.

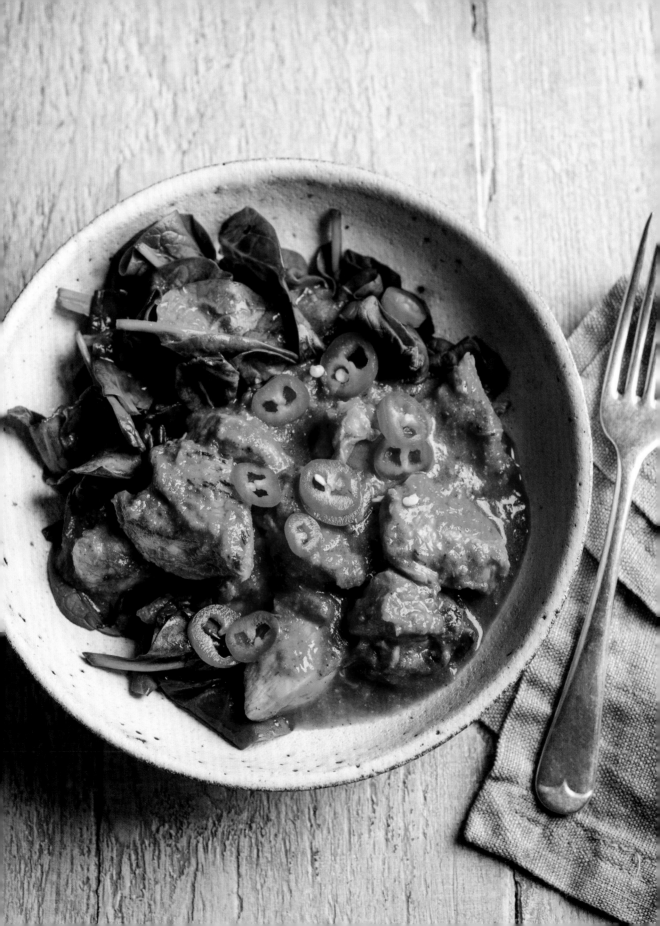

Chicken, pepper and chorizo bake

SERVES 2

1 medium red onion, peeled
   and cut into 12 wedges
4 medium tomatoes, quartered
2 peppers (any colour),
   deseeded and cut into
   roughly 3cm chunks
1 tbsp olive oil
4 boneless, skinless chicken
   thighs (around 400g)
½ tsp hot smoked paprika
25g chorizo, diced

NON-FAST DAYS
Increase the portion size and
add a 400g can of butterbeans,
drained, at the same time
as the chorizo.

A simple chicken bake, full of healthy Mediterranean ingredients and wonderful Spanish flavours. Serve with a large leafy salad.

1 Preheat the oven to 200°C/fan 180°C/Gas 6.

2 Place the onions, tomatoes and peppers in a large baking tray. Drizzle with the oil and toss lightly. Nestle the chicken thighs amongst the vegetables. Sprinkle with paprika, season with sea salt and lots of ground black pepper and roast for 30 minutes.

3 Remove the tray from the oven, add the chorizo and return to the oven for a further 5 minutes, or until the chorizo is hot and beginning to brown.

Easy jerk chicken

SERVES 4

8 boneless, skinless chicken thighs (around 800g)

For the marinade
1 medium onion, peeled and roughly chopped
2 garlic cloves, peeled
1 scotch bonnet chilli or 1 tsp crushed dried chilli flakes
juice 1 large lime, plus extra wedges to serve
2 tbsp dark soy sauce
1 tsp dried thyme
1 tsp ground allspice

NON-FAST DAYS
Swap the lower calorie thigh fillets for bone-in, skin-on thighs. Serve with brown rice cooked in coconut milk and mixed with canned black-eye peas or red kidney beans; Homemade coleslaw (see page 87); or a salsa of tomatoes, avocado, lime and olive oil.

Juicy, spicy Caribbean chicken – ideal for a barbecue and delicious oven-baked, too. Serve with a large mixed salad.

1 Blitz all the marinade ingredients with a good pinch of sea salt and lots of ground black pepper in a food processor to make a paste. Alternatively, grate the onion, crush the garlic and finely chop the chilli before mixing with the remaining ingredients. (Wash your hands well after handling the chilli.) Place the marinade in a large bowl.

2 Carefully score the chicken through the thickest part with a knife. Add the chicken to the marinade, stir well, then cover and leave to marinate in the fridge for at least 2 hours or overnight.

3 Preheat the oven to 200°C/fan 180°C/Gas 6. Line a baking tray with foil.

4 Place the chicken on the prepared tray and brush thickly with the marinade. Cook for 25 minutes, or until lightly browned and cooked through.

5 Serve with lime wedges for squeezing over.

COOK'S TIP

★ If cooking on the barbecue, sear the chicken on both sides over a medium heat then move it to the edges of the barbecue or up on to a higher level to finish cooking more gently for about 25–30 minutes. Turn occasionally and make sure the chicken is cooked through.

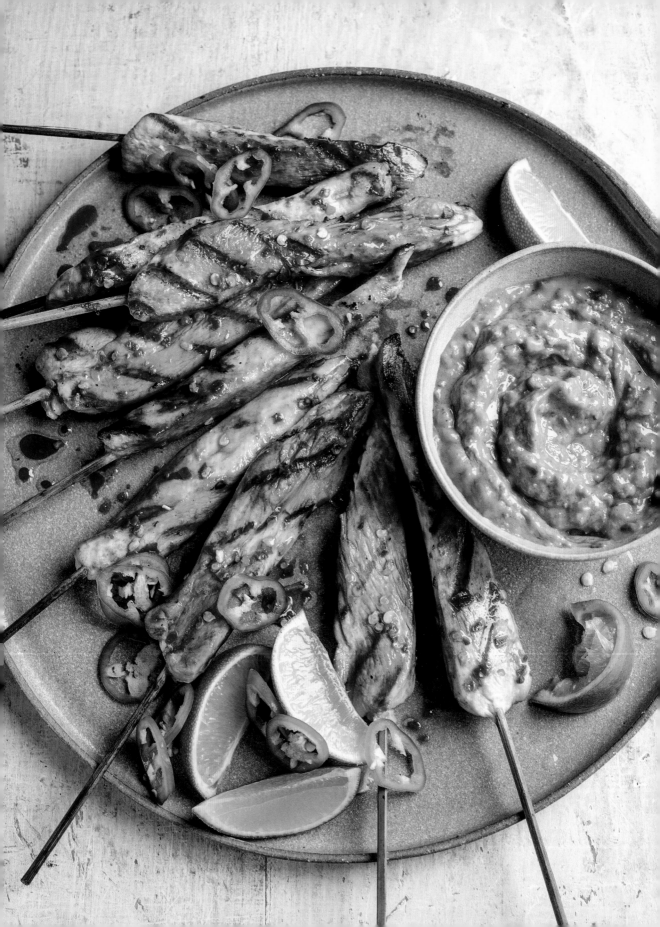

Satay chicken

SERVES 4

1 tbsp coconut or rapeseed oil
juice 1 lime (around 2 tbsp)
½ tsp crushed dried
    chilli flakes
2 tsp dark soy sauce
3 boneless, skinless chicken
    breasts (each around 175g),
    cut into 16 long, thin strips
lime wedges, to serve
1 green chilli, sliced (optional)

For the satay sauce
60g no-added-sugar
    crunchy peanut butter
    (around 4 tbsp)
1 tbsp dark soy sauce
15g fresh root ginger,
    peeled and finely grated

You will need 16 × 20cm bamboo
(soaked in water for 15 minutes)
or metal skewers

NON-FAST DAYS
Increase your portion size
and serve with small portions
of brown rice.

Now that nuts are back on the menu, even on a fast day, you can enjoy this tasty and filling satay sauce as a dip or drizzled. We like cooking these on a ridged griddle, but you can also cook them on the barbecue or under the grill. It's delicious served cold and makes a great portable meal. Serve with a mixed salad.

1 Melt the oil, if using coconut, in a small saucepan very gently then pour into a medium bowl. Add the lime juice, chilli flakes, soy sauce and a good grinding of black pepper. Mix well. Add the chicken strips and toss everything together well.

2 Thread the chicken strips on to the skewers. Work quickly as the lime juice will start 'cooking' the chicken. The coconut oil will also begin to solidify.

3 Place a large lightly greased griddle or non-stick frying pan over a medium–high heat and cook the chicken for 3–4 minutes on each side, depending on thickness, or until lightly browned and cooked through.

4 Meanwhile, to make the satay sauce, place the peanut butter in a small saucepan with around 4 tablespoons water, the soy sauce and grated ginger. Heat gently, stirring constantly until the peanut butter softens and the mixture becomes glossy and thickened. Add a little more soy sauce or water to taste, if needed.

5 Serve the chicken with lime wedges, chilli, if using, and the warm sauce in individual dipping bowls or simply drizzled over.

COOK'S TIP

★ Use metal skewers if cooking on the barbecue or under the grill.

Turkey fajitas

SERVES 4

1 iceberg lettuce
1 tbsp olive or rapeseed oil
400g thin turkey breast steaks,
   cut into thin strips
1 medium red onion, peeled
   and cut into 12 wedges
2 peppers (1 red and 1 yellow),
   deseeded and thinly sliced
1 tsp hot smoked paprika
1 tsp ground cumin
1 tsp ground coriander
handful fresh coriander,
   leaves roughly chopped,
   to serve
100g full-fat live
   Greek yoghurt
lime wedges, to serve

NON-FAST DAYS
Top the turkey with guacamole
and grated cheese, too. Serve in
a small good-quality wholemeal
wrap, if you like.

Turkey makes a fantastic alternative to chicken here
and iceberg lettuce is the perfect carrier for this tasty
Mexican-style filling. Let everyone help themselves
at the table.

1 Turn the lettuce over and cut around the stalk end with
a small knife to separate the leaves. Carefully peel away
at least eight leaves, wash and drain well. Place the leaves
on a board or serving platter.

2 Heat the oil in a large non-stick frying pan over a medium
heat and fry the turkey, onion and peppers for 5–6 minutes,
or until the turkey is cooked and the vegetables are
softened and lightly browned, stirring regularly.

3 Add the spices and cook for 1–2 minutes, stirring. Season
with sea salt and lots of freshly ground black pepper.

4 Take the pan to the table or transfer to a warmed dish
and sprinkle with lots of coriander.

5 Pile the hot turkey into the leaves, top with yoghurt
and serve with lime wedges for squeezing over.

COOK'S TIP

★ Try to avoid the temptation to use a fajita mix, as most
contain added sugars.

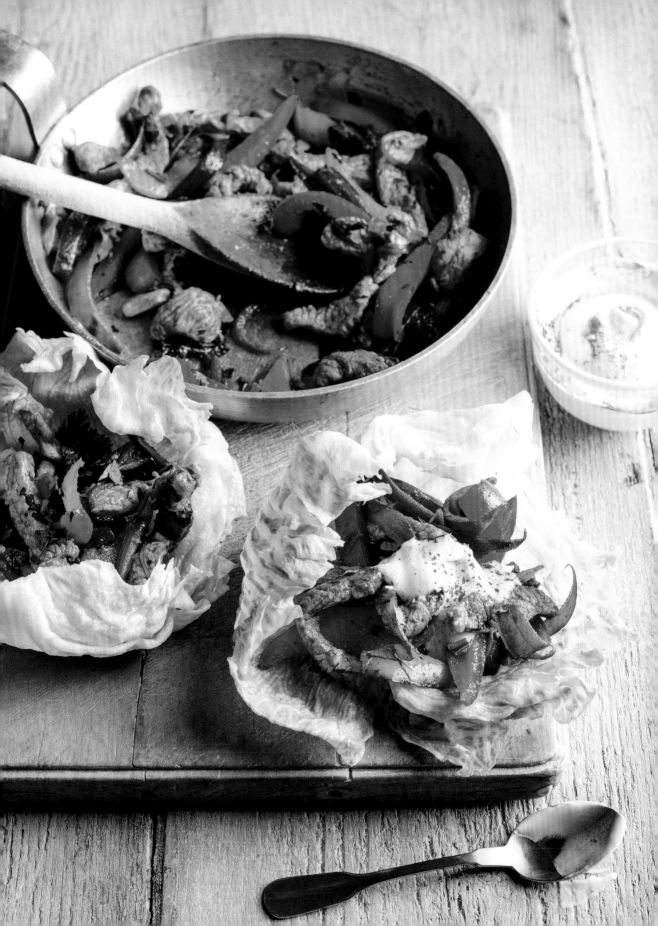

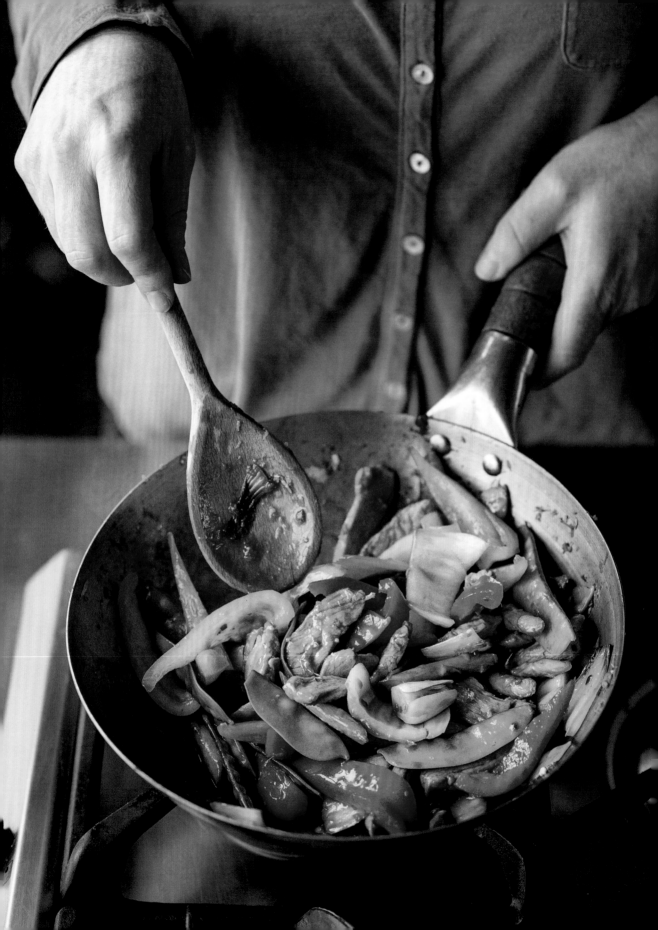

Pork and Ham

Pork is a wonderfully versatile meat and we
have created a good variety of recipes here,
from a Peppered pork stir-fry through a
Courgetti spaghetti with pine nuts, spinach
and pancetta, to a luxurious, slow-cooked
Perfect pulled pork. Try to buy outdoor-
reared if you can.

Perfect pulled pork

SERVES 6

1kg pork shoulder joint,
   trimmed of fat

For the marinade
45g tomato purée
   (around 3 tbsp)
30g chipotle paste
   (around 2 tbsp)
juice 2 medium oranges
juice 2 limes
1 tsp sea salt
1 tsp ground cumin
1 tsp ground allspice
1 tsp ground black pepper

NON-FAST DAYS
Serve in ready-made corn
tacos with lots of salad.

This succulent, zingy pork reheats beautifully, so
can be enjoyed the next day, too. Serve in wraps made
from Little Gem or romaine lettuce leaves topped
with some diced cornichons.

1 To make the marinade, put the tomato purée, chipotle
paste, orange and lime juice, salt and spices in a large
non-metallic bowl and whisk until combined.

2 Remove any string from the pork and add the meat to
the marinade. Turn the pork several times until it is well
coated, then cover and leave to marinate in the fridge for
at least 8 hours or overnight.

3 Preheat the oven to 170°C/fan 150°C/Gas 3.

4 Place the pork and its marinade in a medium casserole,
cover and bake for 3–4 hours, or until the pork falls apart
when prodded with a fork.

5 Transfer the pork to a board or warmed platter and
shred with two forks. Serve with a little of the spicy
cooking juices spooned over.

COOK'S TIPS

★ This goes well with our Homemade coleslaw
(see page 87); or you can buy a good-quality ready-made
coleslaw but don't forget to add the extra calories.
★ You'll find smoky-tasting chipotle chilli paste in the
World Food section of the supermarket, with the Mexican
foods. Or use 2 teaspoons hot smoked paprika instead.
★ If serving fewer people, halve the quantity of pork
and marinade and reduce the cooking time slightly.

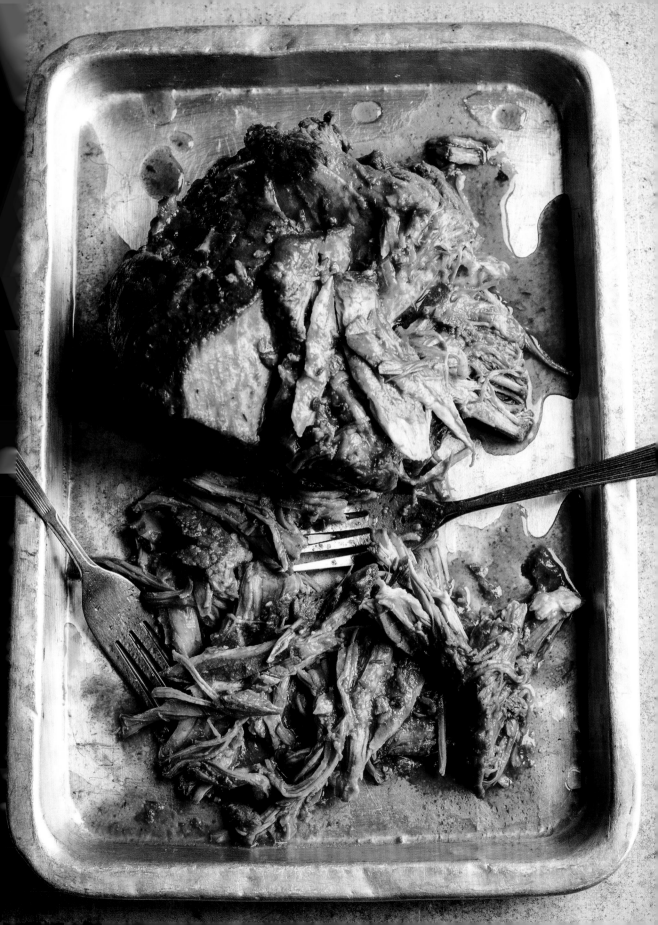

Sausages with onion gravy and cauliflower mash

SERVES 4

2 tsp olive or rapeseed oil

12 good-quality, high-meat chipolata sausages (375g pack)

1 medium onion, peeled and thinly sliced

300ml hot stock (made with ½ pork or ½ chicken stock cube)

2 tbsp reduced sugar tomato ketchup

2 tsp cornflour

For the cauliflower mash

1 medium cauliflower, trimmed, cut into small florets and stalk thinly sliced (700g prepared weight)

1 tbsp olive oil

NON-FAST DAYS

Increase the portion size and add a generous knob of butter or grated mature Cheddar to the cauliflower after blending, and mix well.

Who would believe you could have sausages and mash on a lower carb diet? Our creamy 'mash' is made with cauliflower instead of potatoes, but tastes just as good. Add lots of freshly cooked green vegetables, such as wilted spinach, sliced cabbage or beans.

1 To make the cauliflower mash, half fill a medium pan with water and bring to the boil. Add the cauliflower and return to the boil. Cook for 15–20 minutes or until very soft. Drain, then return to the pan. Add the olive oil, a couple of pinches of sea salt and lots of ground black pepper. Blitz with a stick blender or cool slightly and blend in a food processor until smooth. (You can also mash vigorously with a potato masher.) Keep warm over a very low heat, stirring occasionally.

2 Meanwhile, heat the oil in a large non-stick frying pan and gently fry the sausages for 5 minutes, turning regularly. Add the onion and cook for a further 8–10 minutes, until the sausages are thoroughly cooked and the onion is very soft and lightly browned.

3 Stir in the stock and ketchup and bring to a simmer. Mix the cornflour with 1 tablespoon cold water in a small bowl and stir into the pan. Season well with ground black pepper and simmer for 1–2 minutes, or until thickened and glossy, stirring constantly. Adjust the seasoning to taste.

4 Divide the cauliflower mash between four warmed plates and top with the sausages and gravy.

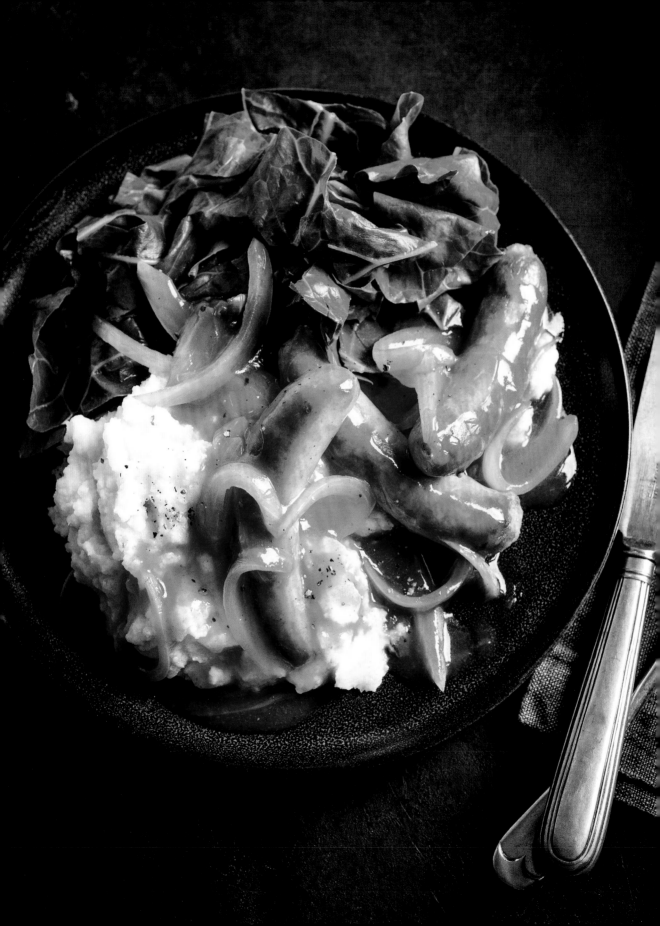

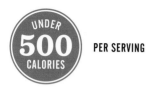

Cheat's one-pot cassoulet

SERVES 4

1 tbsp olive oil
6 spicy sausages
   (around 400g), such as
   Toulouse or spicy pork
1 large onion, peeled
   and thinly sliced
100g cubed smoked lardons,
   pancetta or bacon
1 × 400g can haricot
   or cannellini beans,
   drained and rinsed
1 × 400g can chopped tomatoes
1 tsp dried mixed herbs
generous handful chopped
   fresh parsley, to serve

NON-FAST DAYS
Serve with warmed wholegrain
bread drizzled with olive oil.

This is comfort food from France. Beans, like lentils, are a great source of fibre and have even been found to improve quality of sleep. Serve steaming hot with lots of green leafy vegetables.

1 Heat the oil in a wide-based, non-stick saucepan or flame-proof casserole, add the sausages and cook over a medium heat for about 5 minutes, or until lightly browned on all sides, turning regularly. Remove from the pan and transfer to a board.

2 Add the onion and pancetta to the pan and cook for 3–5 minutes, stirring regularly until golden.

3 Cut the sausages in half and return them to the pan, and add the beans, tomatoes and herbs. Stir in 150ml water and bring to a gentle simmer. Cover loosely and cook for 18–20 minutes, stirring occasionally. Add an extra splash of water if the sauce thickens too much.

4 Season to taste with sea salt and generous amounts of black pepper and stir in the parsley to serve.

COOK'S TIP

★ Look out for full-flavoured sausages for this casserole as they'll add lots of flavour to the sauce. If you can only find the traditional kind, crumble half a chicken stock cube into the sauce, increase the herbs and add ½ teaspoon crushed dried chilli flakes.

Pan-fried pork with apple and leek

SERVES 2

2 pork loin steaks
   (each around 135g)
1 tbsp olive or rapeseed oil
1 small apple, quartered,
   cored and sliced
1 medium leek, trimmed and
   cut into roughly 1cm slices
200ml pork or chicken stock
   (made with ½ stock cube)
1 tsp Dijon or wholegrain
   mustard
45g full-fat crème fraîche
   (around 3 tbsp)

NON-FAST DAYS
Serve with a few tablespoons
of brown rice or swede mash
(see page 180).

A scrumptious, filling pork dish. And one with
prebiotic fibre that your gut microbes will love.
Serve with a large portion of freshly cooked
leafy greens, courgette or green beans.

1 Season the pork on both sides with a little sea salt
and lots of ground black pepper. Heat the oil in a non-stick
frying pan over a medium heat and fry the pork for
3–4 minutes on each side, depending on thickness,
or until lightly browned and cooked through. Don't
overcook or the pork will toughen. Transfer to
a warmed plate.

2 Add the apple and leek to the frying pan and cook
for 2 minutes, or until lightly browned and beginning
to soften.

3 Stir in the stock and mustard and bring to a simmer.
Cook for 3 minutes, or until the leek is soft and the liquid
has reduced by roughly two-thirds, stirring constantly. Stir
in the crème fraîche and cook until melted and bubbling.

4 Return the pork to the pan and warm through for
a minute or two before serving.

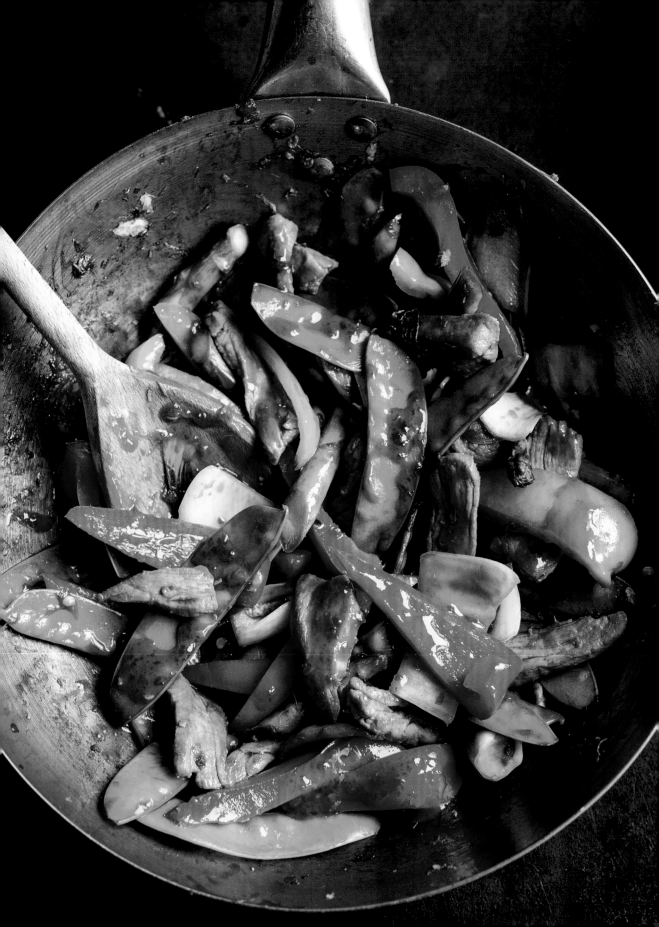

UNDER **300** CALORIES

Peppered pork stir-fry

SERVES 2

250g pork tenderloin
(fillet), trimmed,
cut in half lengthways
then into 1cm slices
1 tbsp coconut or rapeseed oil
1 × 320–350g pack mixed
stir-fry vegetables
15g fresh root ginger,
peeled and finely grated

For the spicy sauce
1 tsp cornflour
1 tbsp dark soy sauce
1 tsp runny honey
¼–½ tsp crushed
dried chilli flakes

NON-FAST DAYS
Add cooked wholewheat or soba
buckwheat noodles and a little
of the noodle water at the same
time as the sauce or serve with
a few tablespoons of brown rice.

A super-quick, super-tasty stir-fry.

1 Season the pork all over with a little sea salt and
a generous amount of freshly ground black pepper.

2 Heat the oil in a large non-stick frying pan or wok
over a medium–high heat. Add the pork and stir-fry,
tossing frequently, for 3–4 minutes, or until lightly
browned and cooked through.

3 Add the vegetables and stir-fry with the pork for
2–3 minutes. Stir in the ginger and cook for a few
seconds more.

4 Meanwhile, for the spicy sauce, mix the cornflour
with the soy sauce, honey and chilli in a small
bowl. Stir into the pan and toss everything together
for 1–2 minutes, or until the vegetables are tender
and glossy. Serve with a little extra soy sauce,
if you like.

COOK'S TIPS

★ Freeze any leftover pork from the whole tenderloin
– wrap tightly in foil and place in the freezer for up
to 3 months.
★ This could also be made with strips of beef, chicken
or tofu. The pork in this recipe contributes 154cals
per serving – adjust the calories accordingly.

PER SERVING | **308cals** | PROTEIN **35g** | FAT **7g** | FIBRE **6g** | CARBS **23.5g**

Parma pork with squash mash

SERVES 3

1kg butternut squash
400g pork tenderloin (fillet),
    trimmed of fat and sinew
3 slices Parma ham or
    prosciutto

NON-FAST DAYS
Serve two rather than three on non-fast days, so each person gets a larger portion.

A gorgeous roast using just three ingredients, with a total preparation time of less than 10 minutes. It also reheats really well, so can be warmed up for lunch or supper the following day. Serve with lots of freshly cooked shredded kale, cabbage or other greens.

1 Preheat the oven to 200°C/fan 180°C/Gas 6 and line a baking tray with foil.

2 Place the whole, unpeeled squash on the baking tray and prick 8–10 times with the tip of a knife. Bake for 1 hour.

3 Meanwhile, wrap the pork in the Parma ham or prosciutto. Place the pork on the tray alongside the squash and return to the oven for a further 25–30 minutes, or until the pork is cooked and the squash is tender. (You should be able to push a knife into the squash easily.)

4 Transfer the pork to a warm plate, cover with foil and leave to rest. Meanwhile, cut the squash in half vertically and, using a large spoon, scoop out and discard the seeds. Scoop the flesh out of the skin and place in a bowl. Season with sea salt and ground black pepper then mash really well.

5 Place the pork on a board, reserving the resting juices, and slice thickly. Spoon the mash on to warmed plates and top with the pork. Drizzle with the juices to serve.

COOK'S TIP

★ Roasted squash makes a great accompaniment to other meals too. The length of cooking time will vary according to the size of the squash. The mashed squash alone contains 55cals per 150g serving.

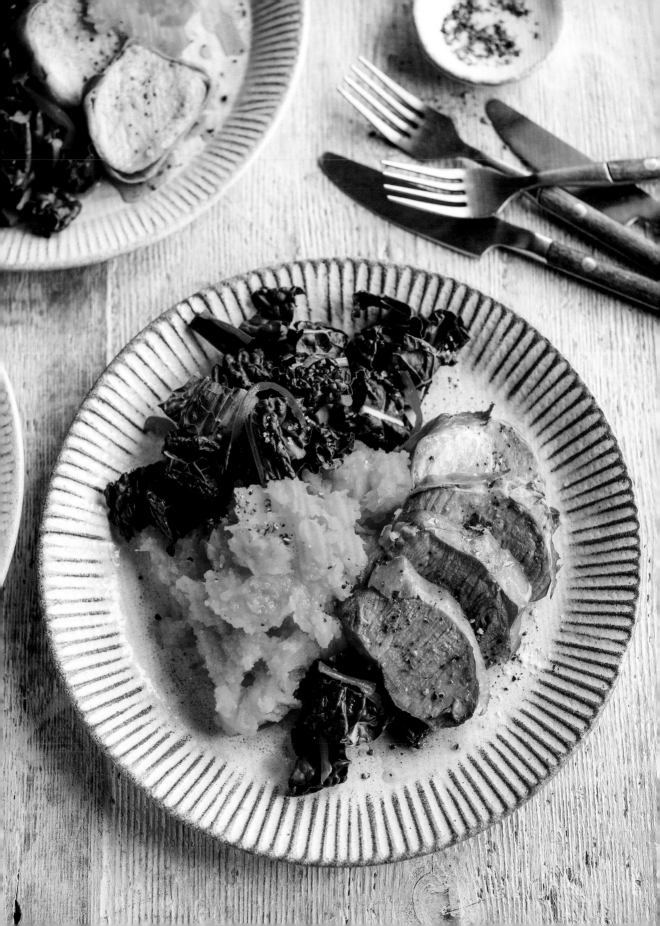

Courgetti spaghetti with pine nuts, spinach and pancetta

SERVES 2

80g dried wholewheat
    spaghetti
1 large courgette, trimmed
    and spiralized (see
    page 242 or 250g ready-
    prepared courgetti)
20g pine nuts
50g cubed smoked lardons or
    pancetta (or diced bacon)
1 tbsp olive oil
150g young spinach leaves
80g feta

NON-FAST DAYS
Increase the amount of
wholewheat spaghetti.

Some token spaghetti gives this delicious carbonara a bit of texture, without adding too many calories. Serve with a salad – use radicchio or red chicory for extra antioxidants.

1 Half fill a large saucepan with water and bring to the boil. Add the spaghetti, return to the boil and cook for 10–12 minutes, or until tender. Add the spiralized courgette and stir together quickly, then immediately strain through a colander, and run very briefly under a cold tap.

2 Meanwhile, place the pine nuts and lardons in a non-stick saucepan with half the oil and fry over a medium heat for 2–3 minutes, stirring regularly until lightly browned. Tip out on to a plate and return the pan to the heat.

3 Add the remaining oil and spinach and cook over a medium heat for 1–2 minutes, or until the spinach is soft, stirring regularly. Crumble two thirds of the feta over the top, season and cook until the feta melts, making a creamy coating for the spinach.

4 Return the spaghetti and courgetti to their saucepan, add the spinach and feta sauce and, using two forks, toss together well over a medium heat for 1–2 minutes.

5 Divide between two shallow bowls, crumble the remaining feta over the top and sprinkle with the pancetta and pine nuts.

COOK'S TIPS

★ If not eating pork, skip the pancetta and reduce the total calories by 60cals per portion.
★ A spiralizer will help to cut courgettes, and other vegetables, into long, thin, spaghetti-like strips. If you don't have one, buy ready-made courgetti. You could also peel the courgette into long strips using a potato peeler.

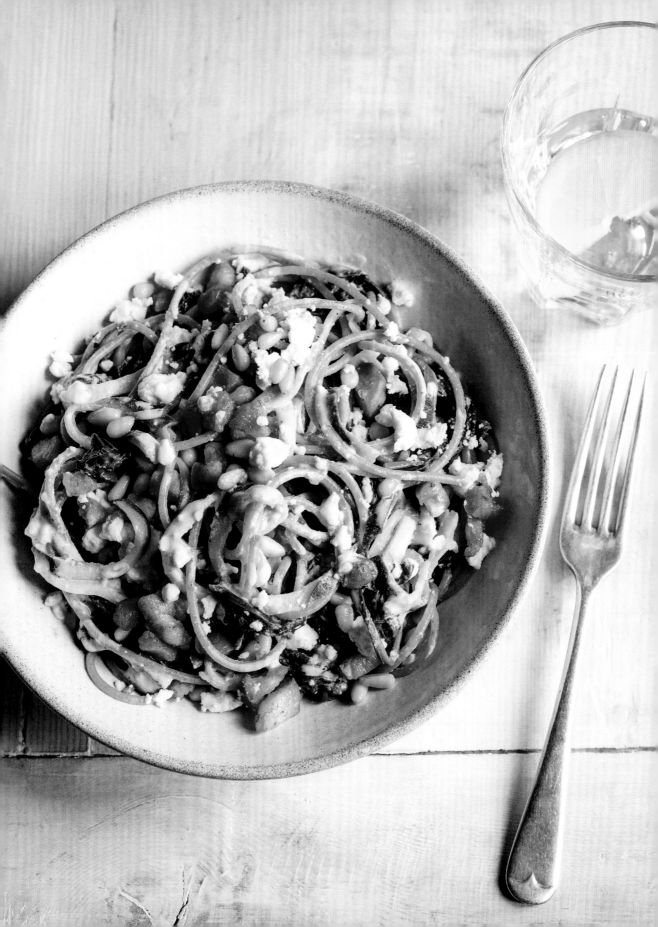

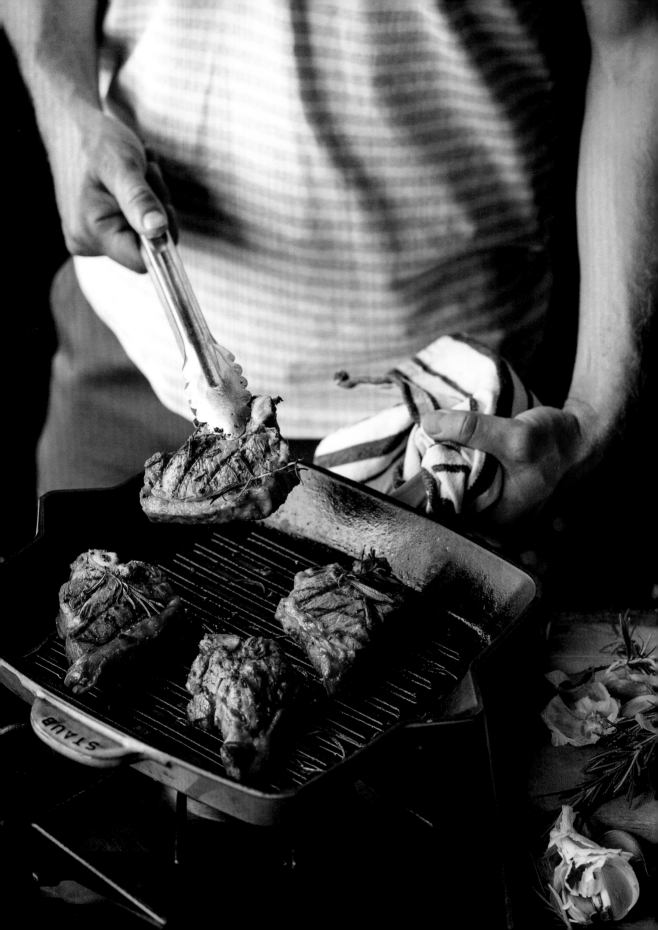

Lamb and Beef

We are generally reducing the amount of red meat we eat, but we love having some in a stew or curry, and every now and then we enjoy a juicy, nutritious steak. These recipes include lamb and beef in moderate quantities, along with lots of lovely vegetables for extra interest and flavour.

Lamb chops with crushed minted peas and feta

SERVES 2

2 thick lamb loin chops
   (each around 175g)
   or 4 lamb cutlets
1 tsp olive oil

*For the crushed minted
peas and feta*
200g frozen peas
1 tbsp olive oil
15g pine nuts, toasted
   (see 84)
1 red chilli, deseeded
   and finely diced
10g fresh mint, leaves
   finely chopped
50g feta

NON-FAST DAYS
Drizzle with more olive oil or
dress the salad with our Simple
salad dressing (see page 241).
Add 2–3 tablespoons of cooked
quinoa or pearl barley.

A quick, easy and wonderfully satisfying supper.
Serve with a leafy salad or a generous portion
of wilted spinach (which tastes even better with
a teaspoon of olive oil or butter – add 40cals).

1 Rub the lamb with the oil and season on both sides
with sea salt and ground black pepper. Heat a griddle,
barbecue or frying pan to a medium–high heat and cook
the chops for 3–5 minutes on each side, depending on
thickness, or until done to taste. Turn on to the fat side
for 30 seconds at the end.

2 Meanwhile, to make the minted peas, third fill a
pan with water and bring to the boil. Add the peas and
cook for 3 minutes. Drain the peas then return to the
pan and mash lightly. Add the olive oil, pine nuts and
chilli, sprinkle with the mint and crumble the feta
on top. Season with lots of ground black pepper
and toss lightly.

3 Divide the lamb and crushed peas between two
plates to serve.

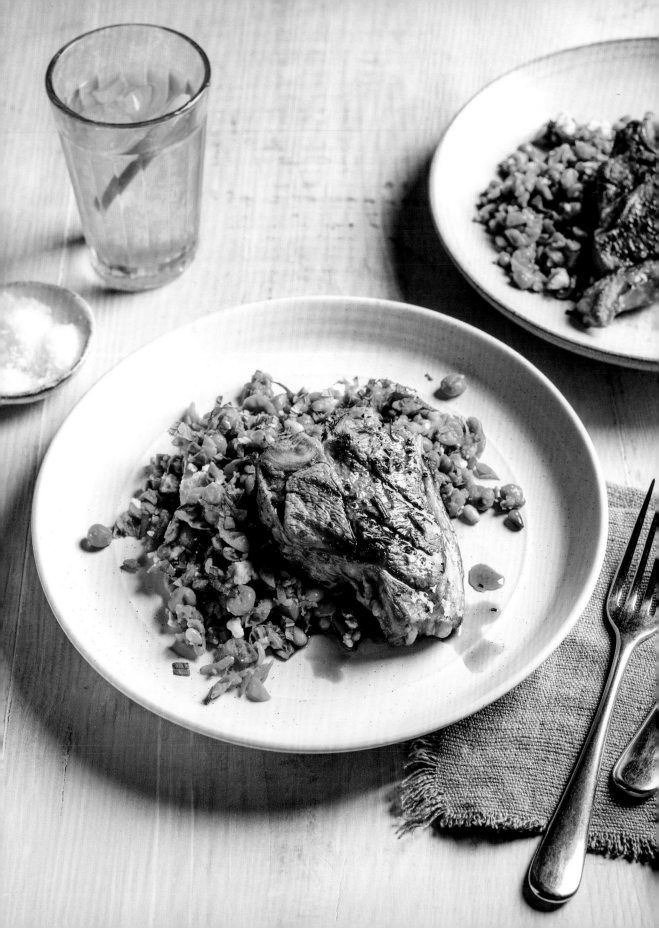

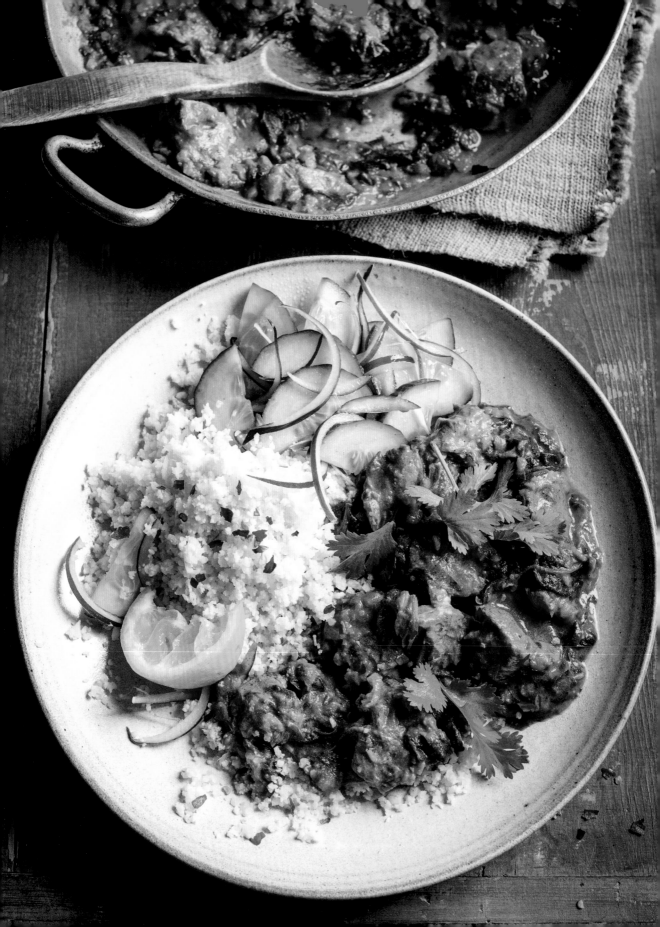

Lamb saag

SERVES 4

1 tbsp coconut or rapeseed oil

1 medium onion, peeled
    and finely sliced

500g lamb neck fillets,
    trimmed and cut into
    roughly 3–4cm chunks

60g (around 4 tbsp) medium
    Indian curry paste, such as
    rogan josh or tikka masala

50g dried red split lentils

200g frozen spinach

NON-FAST DAYS

Enjoy a larger portion. Serve
with a few tablespoonfuls of
brown rice, Minty yoghurt raitha
(see page 106) and pickles.

A handy throw-it-all-together curry that you can bung
in the oven and forget about. Use a good-quality curry
paste for the best results. Serve with cauliflower rice
(see page 242) and a cucumber and red onion salad.

1 Preheat the oven to 180°C/fan 160°C/Gas 4.

2 Heat the oil in a flame-proof casserole and gently fry the
onion for 5 minutes, or until softened and lightly browned.

3 Add the lamb pieces, season with sea salt and ground
black pepper, and cook for 3 minutes, or until coloured
on all sides, turning regularly. Stir in the curry paste
and cook with the lamb and onion for 1 minute.

4 Add the lentils and spinach and stir in 500ml water.
Bring to the boil, cover with a lid and cook in the oven
for 1–1¼ hours, or until the lamb is tender and the
sauce is thick.

Spiced lamb and minted yoghurt

SERVES 2

½ tsp ground cumin

½ tsp ground coriander

2 lean boneless lamb leg steaks
(each around 100g)

2 tbsp olive oil

1 medium red onion, peeled
and cut into 12 wedges

1 pepper (any colour),
deseeded and cut into
roughly 3cm chunks

1 medium courgette, halved
lengthways and cut into
roughly 1.5cm slices

For the minted yoghurt sauce

100g full-fat live Greek
yoghurt

½ small garlic clove,
peeled and crushed

2 tbsp finely chopped
fresh mint leaves

NON-FAST DAYS
Take the lamb steaks out of
the pan once cooked and add
a drained and rinsed 200g can
of chickpeas to the vegetables.
Stir-fry for a couple of
minutes until hot.

**A classic combination of spice-crusted lamb with
colourful Mediterranean vegetables.**

1 Mix the cumin, coriander, a pinch of sea salt and lots
of ground black pepper on a plate. Coat the lamb steaks
on both sides with the spice mix then set aside.

2 To make the minted yoghurt sauce, mix the yoghurt,
garlic and mint in a small bowl and add just enough
cold water to make a drizzly consistency.

3 Heat 1 tablespoon of the oil in a large non-stick frying
pan and gently fry the onion, pepper and courgette for
4–5 minutes, stirring regularly.

4 Push all the vegetables to one side of the pan, add
the remaining 1 tablespoon oil and fry the steaks over
a medium heat for 3–4 minutes on each side, or until
done to taste. (Turn the vegetables occasionally while
the lamb is cooking so they don't burn.)

5 Leave to stand for 5 minutes, then divide between
two plates and drizzle with the yoghurt sauce.

Meatballs in tomato sauce

SERVES 4

300g small good-quality beef
   meatballs (around 20)
1 tbsp olive oil
1 medium onion, peeled
   and finely chopped
2 garlic cloves, peeled
   and crushed
1 × 400g can chopped tomatoes
1 tsp dried oregano
¼–½ tsp crushed dried
   chilli flakes (optional)

5:2

NON-FAST DAYS
Serve the Mediterranean
meatballs with small portions
of wholegrain pasta, or bean,
lentil or pea pasta and sprinkle
with a little grated Parmesan.
Serve the Moroccan version
with a few tablespoons of
quinoa or brown rice.

You can make this dish with the classic Mediterranean
flavours suggested here, or give it a more exotic
Moroccan taste (see cook's tip). Serve with a large
helping of lightly cooked courgetti (see page 242)
and a leafy salad.

1 Preheat the oven to 200°C/fan 180°C/Gas 6.

2 Place the meatballs on a baking tray and cook for
10 minutes.

3 Meanwhile, for the tomato sauce, heat the oil in a large
non-stick frying pan and gently fry the onion for 5 minutes,
or until softened and lightly browned, stirring regularly.
Add the garlic and cook for a few seconds more, stirring.

4 Tip the tomatoes into the pan, add 200ml water, the
oregano and chilli, if using, and bring to a gentle simmer.
Cook for 5 minutes, stirring.

5 Remove the meatballs from the oven and transfer to the
tomato sauce. Season with sea salt and ground black pepper
and cook for a further 5 minutes, or until the meatballs are
thoroughly cooked. Stir regularly and add a splash of water
if the sauce thickens too much.

COOK'S TIP

★ For a **Moroccan-style version of the recipe**, with
300cals per serving, fry the onion with 1 diced pepper
for 5 minutes then add 1 teaspoon ground cumin and fry
for a few seconds before adding 1 tablespoon harissa paste
and 6 quartered dried apricots as well as the tomatoes,
water, oregano and chilli. Finish with a generous
scattering of freshly chopped coriander.

PER SERVING | **346cals** | PROTEIN **30g** | FAT **22g** | FIBRE **3g** | CARBS **5g**

Simple steak and salad

SERVES 2

225g lean sirloin beef
    steak, cut in half
1 tbsp olive oil
150g button chestnut
    mushrooms, halved
    or sliced if large

For the salad
100g mixed leaves
½ yellow pepper,
    deseeded and sliced
10 cherry tomatoes, halved
⅓ cucumber (around 135g),
    sliced
2 spring onions, trimmed
    and finely sliced

For the balsamic dressing
2 tbsp extra-virgin olive oil
2 tsp balsamic vinegar

A juicy steak with a colourful dressed salad is
a fantastic, easy, low-carb combination, which
provides a good protein boost on a fast day.

1 To make the salad, toss all the ingredients in a bowl.

2 Season the beef all over with sea salt and lots of
ground black pepper.

3 Heat the oil in a large non-stick frying pan over a
medium–high heat and fry the steaks for 3–4 minutes
on each side, or until done to taste. Place the steaks
on two warmed plates and leave to rest.

4 Add the mushrooms to the pan and cook for
2–3 minutes, or until browned, stirring regularly.
Spoon on top of the steaks.

5 Drizzle the oil and vinegar over the salad and toss
lightly. Serve alongside the steak and mushrooms.

NON-FAST DAYS
Serve with roasted butternut
squash wedges, add a generous
spoonful of full-fat crème
fraîche to the mushrooms
just before the end of their
cooking time and double up
the dressing ingredients.

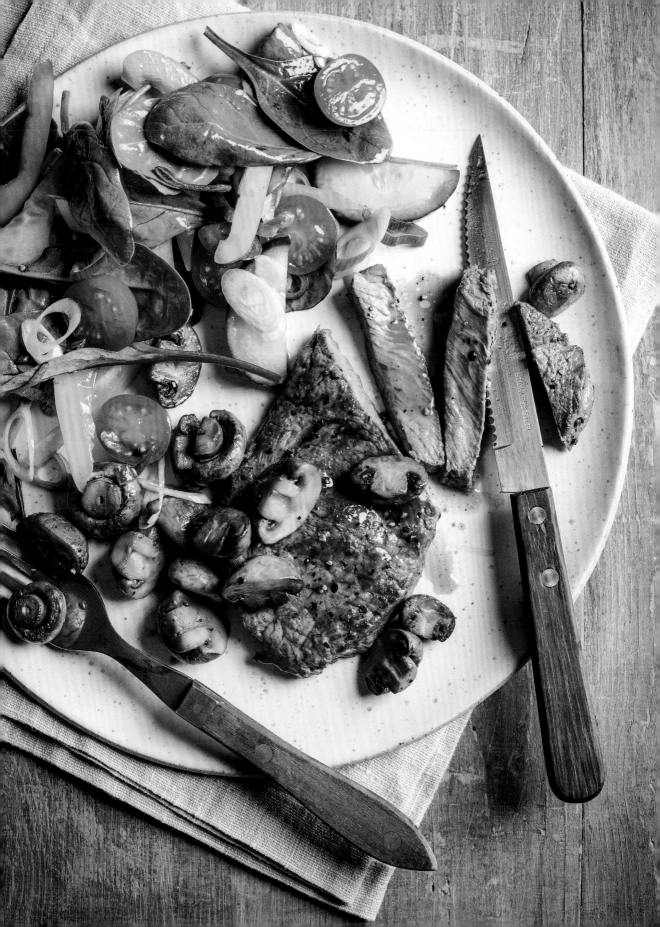

PER SERVING | **354cals** | PROTEIN **27g** | FAT **16g** | FIBRE **10g** | CARBS **21g**

Cottage pie with swede mash

SERVES 5

2 tbsp olive oil

500g lean minced beef (around 10% fat)

1 medium onion, peeled and finely chopped

200g carrots (around 2 medium), trimmed and cut into roughly 1cm chunks

1 beef stock cube

2 tbsp tomato purée

1 tbsp Worcestershire sauce

1 tsp dried mixed herbs

1.2kg swede (around 1 large or 2 small), peeled and cut into roughly 3cm chunks

150g frozen peas

NON-FAST DAYS

Mix the mashed swede with full-fat crème fraîche or grated mature Cheddar, or a good slug of olive oil.

A family favourite given a low-carb make-over. Eat leftovers another day or freeze them. Serve with lots of freshly cooked green vegetables.

1 Heat the oil in a large non-stick saucepan and gently fry the mince, onion and carrots for 8–10 minutes, or until the mince is browned and the onions softened.

2 Crumble the stock cube over the mince and stir in 700ml water, the tomato purée, Worcestershire sauce and herbs. Bring to a simmer and season generously with sea salt and ground black pepper. Cover loosely and cook for about 25 minutes, stirring occasionally, adding a little more water, if needed. The mince should be tender and fairly saucy.

3 Preheat the oven to 220°C/fan 200°C/Gas 7.

4 Meanwhile, to make the swede mash, place the swede in a large saucepan and fill with cold water. Cover with a lid and bring to the boil. Cook for 20 minutes, or until soft. Drain the swede in a colander then return to the pan and mash with a potato masher until as smooth as possible. Season with sea salt and ground black pepper.

5 Add the frozen peas to the mince and cook for 1 minute, stirring constantly. Pour carefully into a 2-litre shallow ovenproof dish. Spoon the swede on top of the mince and bake for 25–30 minutes, or until the swede is tipped with brown and the filling is bubbling. (It won't go golden like mashed potato.)

Beef stroganoff

SERVES 2
250g sirloin steak
2 tbsp olive or rapeseed oil
1 medium onion, peeled
　and thinly sliced
150g button chestnut
　mushrooms, sliced
1 tsp paprika (not smoked)
175ml beef stock (made
　with ½ beef stock cube)
2 tsp cornflour
30g (around 2 tbsp)
　full-fat crème fraîche
chopped fresh parsley,
　to serve

5:2

NON-FAST DAYS
Serve with brown or wild rice
and extra crème fraîche.

This tasty, satisfying beef dish includes lots of lovely mushrooms, which add extra taste and texture with minimal calories. Serve with cauliflower rice (see page 242) or courgetti (see page 242) and a mixed side salad.

1 Trim any fat from the steak and cut on a slight diagonal into long thin strips, not more than 1cm wide. Season well with sea salt and ground black pepper.

2 Heat 1 tablespoon of the oil in a large non-stick frying pan over a medium–high heat. Add the steak and fry for 2–3 minutes, or until browned but not cooked through. Tip the beef on to a plate and return the pan to the heat.

3 Add the remaining oil to the pan with the onion and mushrooms, and cook for 4–5 minutes, or until the onions are softened and lightly browned. Sprinkle with paprika and cook for a few seconds more.

4 Pour the stock into the pan and bring to a simmer. Cook for 2 minutes, stirring regularly.

5 Mix the cornflour with 1 tablespoon cold water in a small bowl and stir into the pan. Add the crème fraîche and return the beef to the pan. Warm the beef in the sauce for 1–2 minutes, adding an extra splash of water if needed, stirring regularly. Sprinkle with chopped fresh parsley to serve.

COOK'S TIP

★ You can make this with strips of chicken or turkey breast instead, but remember to adjust the calories: 200g sirloin steak contains 268cals; 200g chicken breast 212cals; and 200g turkey breast 210cals.

PER SERVING | **259cals** | PROTEIN **24g** | FAT **13.5g** | FIBRE **8g** | CARBS **6g**

Classic burger with celeriac chips

SERVES 4

½ medium onion,
   peeled and coarsely grated
   or very finely chopped
1 garlic clove, peeled
   and finely grated
100g carrot (around
   1 medium), trimmed
   and finely grated
400g lean minced beef
   (around 10% fat)
½ tsp flaked sea salt
½ tsp dried mixed herbs

For the celeriac chips
750g celeriac, peeled (around
   600g peeled weight)
1 tbsp olive or rapeseed oil

5:2

NON-FAST DAYS
Top the burgers with slices
of blue cheese and pop under
the grill. Add spoonfuls of
our Homemade coleslaw
(see page 87) if you like.

Adding grated carrot to burgers makes them extra juicy and boosts the fibre. And with this low-carb recipe you still get to munch your chips. Serve the burgers with a large mixed salad.

1 Preheat the oven to 220°C/fan 200°C/Gas 7.

2 To make the celeriac chips, carefully cut the celeriac into roughly 1.5cm slices and then into chips. Place in a bowl with the oil, a couple pinches of sea salt and lots of ground black pepper. Toss well together. Scatter over a baking tray and bake for 20 minutes. Turn the chips and return to the oven for a further 5–10 minutes, or until tender and lightly browned.

3 Meanwhile, make the burgers. Put the onion, garlic, carrot, mince, salt and dried mixed herbs in a bowl, season with lots of ground black pepper and combine thoroughly with your hands.

4 Divide the mixture into 4 balls and flatten into burger shapes. Make them a little flatter than you think they should be, as they will shrink as they cook.

5 Place a large non-stick frying pan over a medium heat and cook the burgers without any additional fat for 10 minutes, or until lightly browned and cooked through, turning occasionally. Press the burgers every now and then with a spatula so they cook evenly.

6 Divide the chips between four warmed plates and serve a burger alongside.

COOK'S TIP

★ We use a few cherry tomatoes in the salad for colour, but any more than that and you would need to include the calories if you are on a fast day.

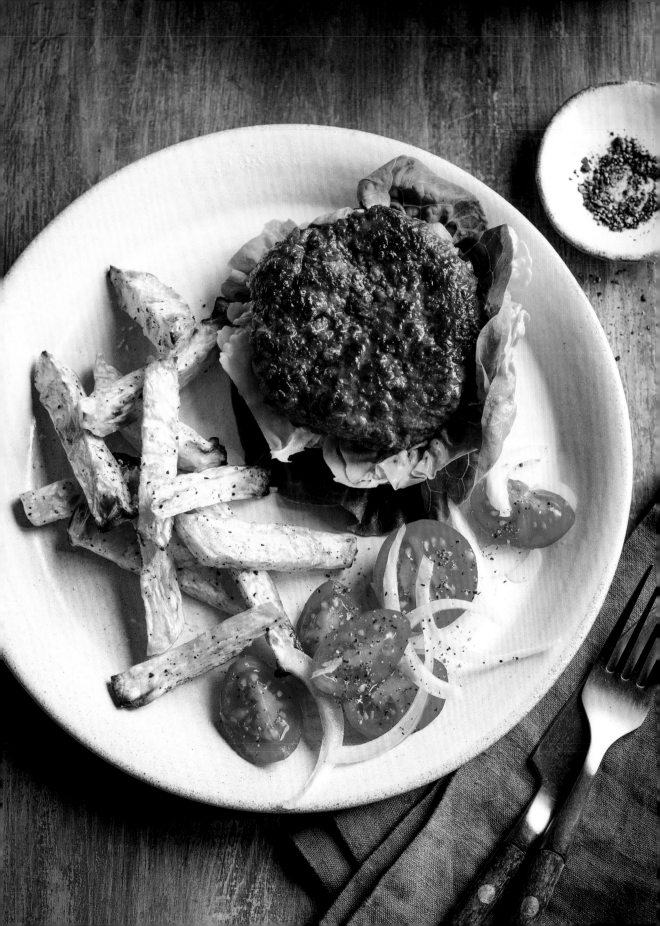

| PER SERVING | **482cals** | PROTEIN **36g** | FAT **31.5g** | FIBRE **2.5g** | CARBS **12.5g**

Beef rendang

SERVES 4

600g beef braising steak,
trimmed and cut into
roughly 4cm chunks
6 garlic cloves, peeled
50g fresh root ginger, peeled
and roughly chopped
2 medium red onions,
peeled and quartered
1 tsp crushed dried chilli flakes
2 tbsp coconut or rapeseed oil
1 × 400ml can coconut milk
3 tbsp dark soy sauce
1 beef stock cube
½ tsp ground cinnamon
2 stalks lemongrass,
trimmed (optional)
lime wedges, to serve

NON-FAST DAYS
Serve with 2–3 tablespoons
of cooked brown rice and
some Minty yoghurt raitha
(see page 106).

This recipe is a pared down version of the Malaysian
classic but is incredibly delicious and satisfying. Serve
with steamed spring greens, long-stemmed broccoli
or pak choi.

1 Preheat the oven to 170°C/fan 150°C/Gas 3. Season the
beef with a sea salt and lots of freshly ground black pepper.

2 Put the garlic, ginger, onions and chilli flakes in a food
processor and blitz until very finely chopped.

3 Heat 1 tablespoon of the oil in a large non-stick frying
pan over a high heat. Fry the beef in two batches until
lightly browned on all sides and transfer to a flame-proof
casserole dish.

4 Add the remaining oil to the pan and gently fry the garlic
and onion mixture for 5 minutes, stirring constantly.

5 Add to the casserole with the beef and stir in the
coconut milk, soy sauce and 200ml water. Crumble in
the stock cube and add the cinnamon. If using lemongrass,
snap each stalk twice without completely separating the
pieces, or bash with a rolling pin, and add to the curry
(this will release their flavour). Stir well and bring to
a simmer. Cover with a lid and cook in the oven for
2¾–3¼ hours, or until the beef is meltingly tender.

COOK'S TIPS

★ Lemongrass stalks can be found with the garlic and
ginger in the supermarket, but you can use a couple of
tablespoons of puréed lemongrass from a jar if you prefer.
★ If you don't have a food processor, grate the garlic, ginger
and onion. You could also simplify the recipe by using a
ready-made rendang paste, but these tend to contain sugar.

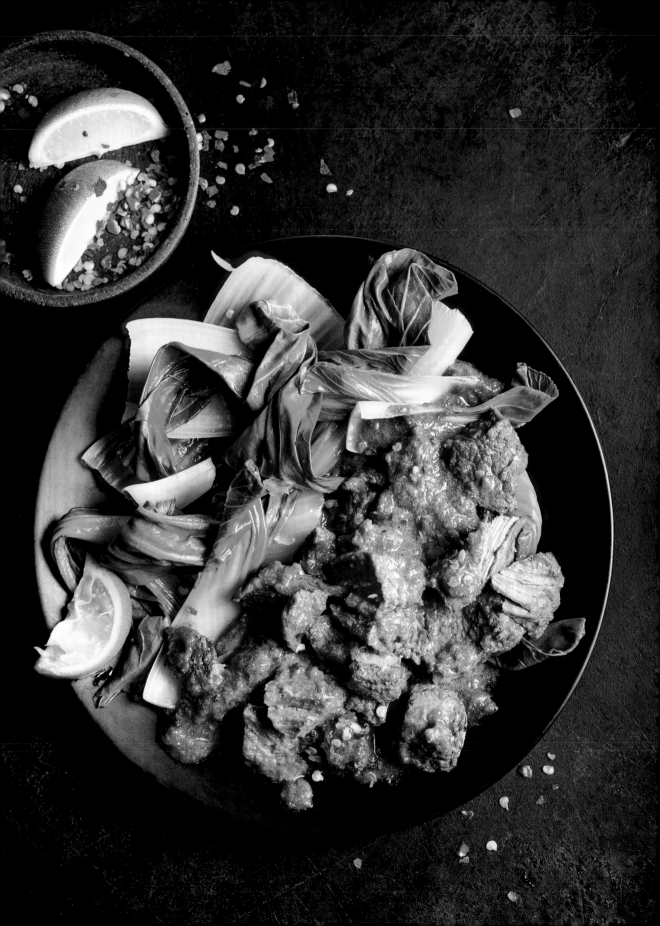

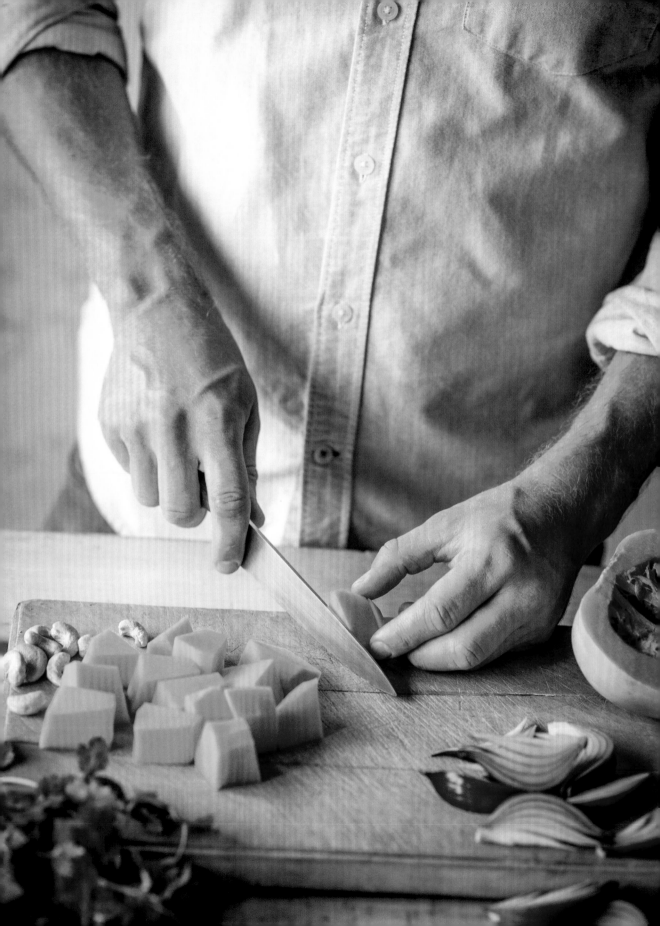

Meat-free

These recipes are mainly plant-based –
some contain dairy or eggs, added for
flavour and to boost protein intake
on fasting days – and they can be
supplemented by a number of recipes
in the meat chapters, where we suggest
vegetarian swaps to offer more options.
The extra fibre of a more vegetable-based
diet will help your good bacteria thrive –
although, if you are not used to a higher
fibre diet, you might want to adjust to
it slowly at first. And don't forget to be
generous with healthy, plant-based
fats, such as olive oil.

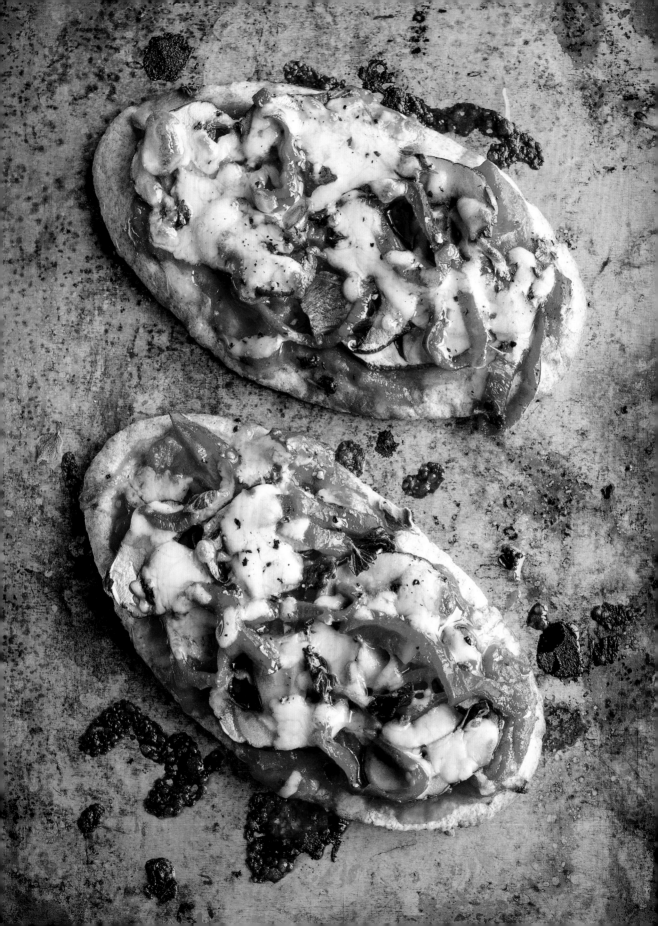

Speedy pizza

SERVES 2

1 × 227g can chopped tomatoes
(or ½ × 400g can)

1 tbsp tomato purée

½ tsp dried oregano,
or a few roughly chopped
fresh oregano leaves

1 wholemeal pitta bread
(around 58g)

2 roasted red peppers
from a jar (around 40g),
drained and sliced

2 chestnut mushrooms
(around 45g),
very finely sliced

35g ready-grated mozzarella

1 tbsp extra-virgin olive oil

NON-FAST DAYS
Make using a whole pitta per
serving and add pitted olives
and a sprinkling of pine nuts.
For a meat version, top the pizza
with sliced salami or chorizo.
Add a dressing to the salad.

**The perfect wholegrain pizza also happens to
be the quickest! Serve with a large mixed salad.**

1 Preheat the grill to a medium-hot setting.

2 To make the pizza topping, tip the tomatoes into a sieve
and shake to remove the excess juice. (There's no need
to press it.) Transfer the tomato pulp to a bowl and stir
in the tomato purée and oregano. Season with a pinch
of sea salt and lots of ground black pepper.

3 Lightly toast the pitta bread, just enough to warm it up,
then place on a board and carefully cut the bread in half
horizontally with a bread knife and separate the two oval
pieces. Place them on a baking tray, cut side down.

4 Spread the pitta halves with the tomato sauce and top
with the peppers, mushrooms and mozzarella. Drizzle
with the olive oil and place under the grill for 4–5 minutes,
or until the cheese has melted and the tomato topping,
mushrooms and peppers are hot.

COOK'S TIPS

★ Ready-grated mozzarella comes in bags and is great
for making pizzas. Use for toppings and sauces and
freeze any that you won't use up in a couple of days.

★ For extra protein, anchovies or chorizo can be
added, if you have spare calories (see page 240).

Baked Camembert with pears and chicory

SERVES 4

1 × 250g round Camembert
   in a box
25g walnut or pecan halves
1 tsp runny honey
2 firm but ripe pears,
   cored and cut into wedges
2 red or white heads chicory,
   leaves separated,
   or assorted vegetable sticks
small handful fresh thyme
   leaves (optional)

NON-FAST DAYS
Serve as a starter instead
of a main meal.

A glorious way to serve Camembert, either as a hassle-free, low-carb lunch or as a dip for sharing.

1 Preheat the oven to 200°C/fan 180°C/Gas 6.

2 Take the Camembert out of its wooden box and remove the wrapping. Place on a board and, holding it on its side, carefully cut the top layer of rind off. Put back in the box, without any wrapping, rind side down. (Transfer to an ovenproof dish if cooking in a gas oven or if the cheese hasn't come packed in a wooden box.) Place on a small baking tray.

3 Roughly chop the nuts and sprinkle on top of the cheese. Drizzle the honey over – this will make the nuts lovely and crunchy – and season with lots of ground black pepper. Bake uncovered for about 15 minutes, or until the cheese is melted and gooey.

4 Serve the melted cheese on a platter with the thyme scattered over the top, surrounded with the pear and chicory or vegetable sticks.

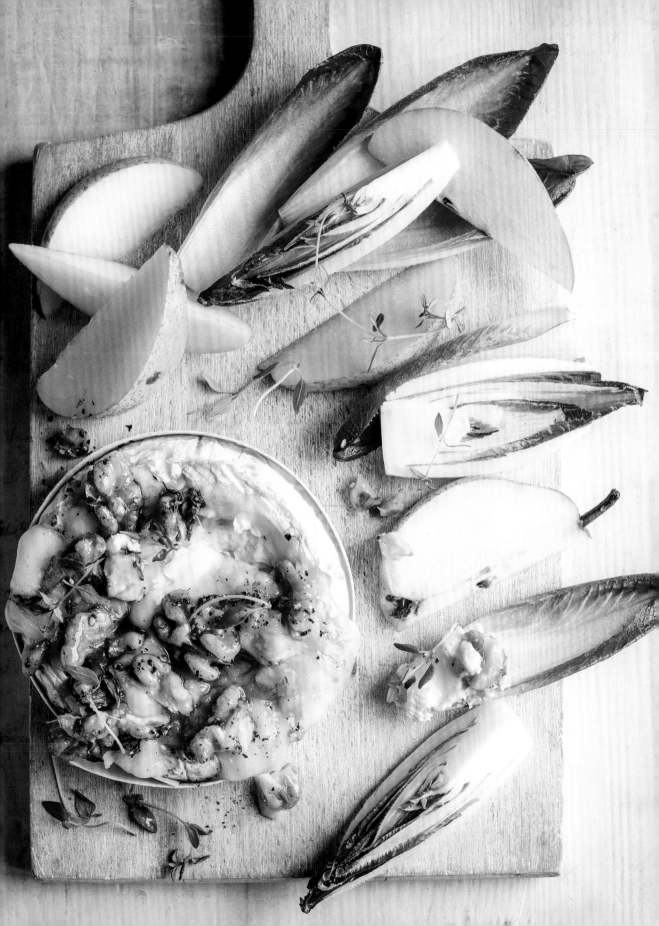

PER SERVING | **346cals** | PROTEIN **18g** | FAT **17g** | FIBRE **10g** | CARBS **26g**

Spicy bean chilli

SERVES 4

2 tbsp olive oil

1 medium onion, peeled
   and thinly sliced

1–1½ tsp hot smoked paprika
   (to taste)

1 tsp ground cumin

1 tsp ground coriander

1 × 400g can chopped tomatoes

1 × 400g can black beans or
   red kidney beans, drained

1 × 400g can mixed
   beans, drained

300ml vegetable stock
   (made with 1 stock cube)

1 tbsp tomato purée

1 tsp dried oregano
   or mixed dried herbs

75g mature Cheddar, grated

100g full-fat live
   Greek yoghurt

NON-FAST DAYS

Serve with brown rice and
top with sliced avocado. Drizzle
the salad with our Simple salad
dressing (see page 241), or
a splash of balsamic vinegar
and glug of olive oil.

A rich, spicy chilli made with a mixture of different
beans to give you plenty of fibre and slow-release
complex carbs. Your microbiome will love it, too.
Serve with a large mixed salad.

1 Heat the oil in a large, deep, non-stick frying pan,
wide-based saucepan or shallow flame-proof casserole,
and gently fry the onion for 3–4 minutes, or until
softened, stirring frequently.

2 Add the smoked paprika, cumin and coriander and
cook for a few seconds, stirring.

3 Add the tomatoes, beans, vegetable stock, tomato purée
and dried herbs, season with sea salt and lots of ground
black pepper and bring to a simmer. Cover loosely with
a lid and cook for 15–20 minutes, or until the sauce has
reduced and thickened, stirring occasionally.

4 Serve topped with the Cheddar and generous spoonfuls
of Greek yoghurt.

COOK'S TIPS

★ If you have IBS, you might need to reduce the bean
portions or skip this recipe.

★ For extra depth of flavour, add a tablespoon of cocoa
powder (11cals per serving) along with the dried herbs.

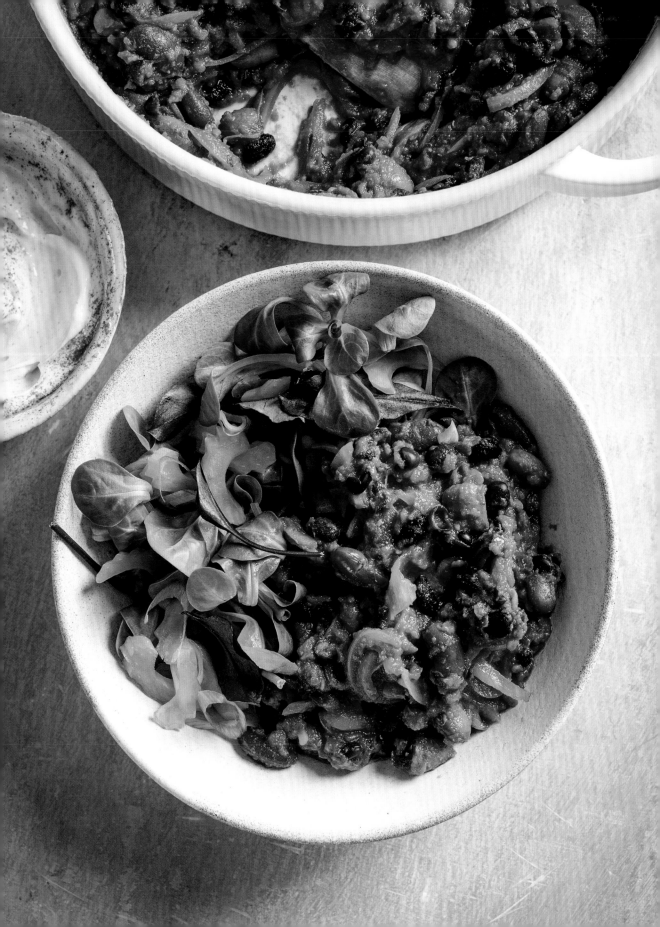

PER SERVING | **207cals** | PROTEIN **12.5g** | FAT **8.5g** | FIBRE **8g** | CARBS **16g**

Dan's veggie Bolognese

SERVES 4

1 red pepper, deseeded
    and cut into roughly
    2cm chunks
1 medium carrot,
    trimmed and cut into
    roughly 1.5cm chunks
3 tbsp olive oil
2 medium onions, peeled
    and finely chopped
2 sticks celery, trimmed
    and thinly sliced
150g small chestnut
    mushrooms, sliced
300g frozen Quorn mince
75g dried red split lentils
1 large garlic clove,
    peeled and crushed
2 × 400g cans chopped
    tomatoes
1 tsp dried oregano
1 vegetable stock cube

NON-FAST DAYS
Serve with wholewheat
spaghetti, allowing roughly
60g dried pasta per person.
Sprinkle with grated Parmesan
and serve with a large, lightly
dressed mixed leaf and
avocado salad. Try pea,
bean or lentil pasta for
a gluten-free alternative.

This Bolognese tastes really rich but is surprisingly low in calories. It was cooked for us by our son Dan and has become a favourite. By baking the vegetables first, their flavour and texture is deliciously enhanced. Serve with freshly cooked courgetti (see page 242).

1 Preheat the oven to 220°C/fan 200°C/Gas 7.

2 Place the pepper and carrot on a baking tray and drizzle with 1 tablespoon of the olive oil. Season with sea salt and ground black pepper and toss lightly. Bake for 15–20 minutes, or until softened and lightly browned.

3 Meanwhile, heat the remaining oil in a deep frying pan or shallow flame-proof casserole and gently fry the onions, celery and mushrooms for 10 minutes, stirring regularly.

4 Add the Quorn mince, lentils and garlic, and cook for 2 minutes more, stirring.

5 Tip the tomatoes into the pan, sprinkle with the oregano and crumble over the stock cube. Add 300ml water, bring to a simmer and cook for 5 minutes, stirring occasionally.

6 Remove the tray from the oven and transfer the roasted vegetables to the pan. Return to a gentle simmer and cook for a further 15 minutes, or until the sauce is thick, stirring regularly. Adjust the seasoning to taste.

COOK'S TIP

★ Sprinkle each portion with 10g freshly grated Parmesan for an extra 41cals per serving.

Mushroom and vegetable biryani

SERVES 4

2 tbsp olive oil

1 medium onion, peeled
and thinly sliced

200g chestnut mushrooms,
thinly sliced

4 medium eggs, fridge cold

2 tbsp medium Indian curry
paste, such as tikka
masala or rogan josh

400g pack frozen mixed
vegetables, such as
peas, broccoli, carrots
and cauliflower

200ml vegetable stock
(made with 1 stock cube)

250g pouch ready-cooked
brown/wholegrain rice

25g flaked almonds, toasted
(see page 18)

handful fresh coriander,
leaves roughly chopped

NON-FAST DAYS
Increase the portion size.

A filling, meat-free, midweek meal. We love mushrooms
– leave them in the sunlight and they produce even
more vitamin D. Choose a good-quality curry paste
from the World Foods section of the supermarket;
it will keep for several weeks in the fridge.

1 Heat the oil in a large, non-stick, wide-based saucepan
or shallow flame-proof casserole over a medium–high heat,
and fry the onion and mushrooms for 5–6 minutes, stirring
regularly, until lightly browned.

2 Half fill a pan with water and bring to the boil. Add the
eggs and return to the boil. Cook for 9 minutes. Drain the
eggs and rinse under cold water until they are cool enough
to handle. Peel and cut into quarters.

3 Stir the curry paste into the pan with the onion and
mushrooms and cook for 1 minute, stirring. Add the frozen
vegetables and stock. Bring the liquid to a simmer and
cook for 5 minutes, or until the vegetables are tender,
stirring regularly.

4 Add the rice to the curried vegetables and cook for about
3 minutes more, or until steaming hot, stirring regularly.

5 Place the eggs on top and heat through without stirring
for 1–2 minutes. Sprinkle with the almonds and coriander
to serve.

COOK'S TIP

★ For a non-veggie alternative, slice 2 chicken breasts
and fry with the onion and mushrooms in step 1 (add
an extra 80cals per serving).

Creamy cashew and tofu curry

SERVES 4

2 tbsp coconut or rapeseed oil

1 medium aubergine
  (around 225g), cut into
  roughly 2cm chunks

1 medium red onion, peeled
  and cut into 12 wedges

350g butternut squash,
  peeled, deseeded and cut
  into roughly 2cm chunks

4 tbsp Thai red or
  green curry paste

1 × 400ml can full-fat
  coconut milk

100g cashew nuts,
  roughly chopped

1 large pepper (any colour),
  deseeded and cut into
  roughly 2cm chunks

20g fresh coriander, leaves
  roughly chopped

280g firm, or extra-firm
  tofu, drained, cut into
  roughly 2cm cubes

300g cauliflower rice
  (see page 242; optional)

NON-FAST DAYS
Serve with a small portion
of brown rice or wholewheat
noodles.

Thai-style curries always seem to go down well and
this one is low on carbs and high in flavour. If you don't
like tofu, try Quorn pieces instead. Please note, some
curry pastes contain fish sauce.

1 Heat 1 tablespoon of the oil in a large pan or shallow
casserole over a high heat. Add the aubergine and stir-fry
for 4–5 minutes, until golden brown. Transfer to a bowl.

2 Reduce the heat, add the remaining oil, onion and squash
to the pan and fry gently for 5 minutes, stirring regularly.
Add the curry paste and cook for 1 minute, stirring constantly.

3 Stir in the coconut milk, half the nuts, the pepper and
100ml water. Season with sea salt and ground black pepper.
Cover the pan loosely with a lid, bring to a gentle simmer
and cook for 10 minutes, stirring occasionally.

4 Stir the aubergine and half the coriander into the pan
and return to a simmer. Add the tofu, cover and cook for
a further 5–6 minutes, until the aubergine is softened and
the tofu hot. Add a splash more water if the curry reduces
too much.

5 Sprinkle with the reserved coriander and cashew nuts,
and serve with freshly cooked cauliflower rice, if using.

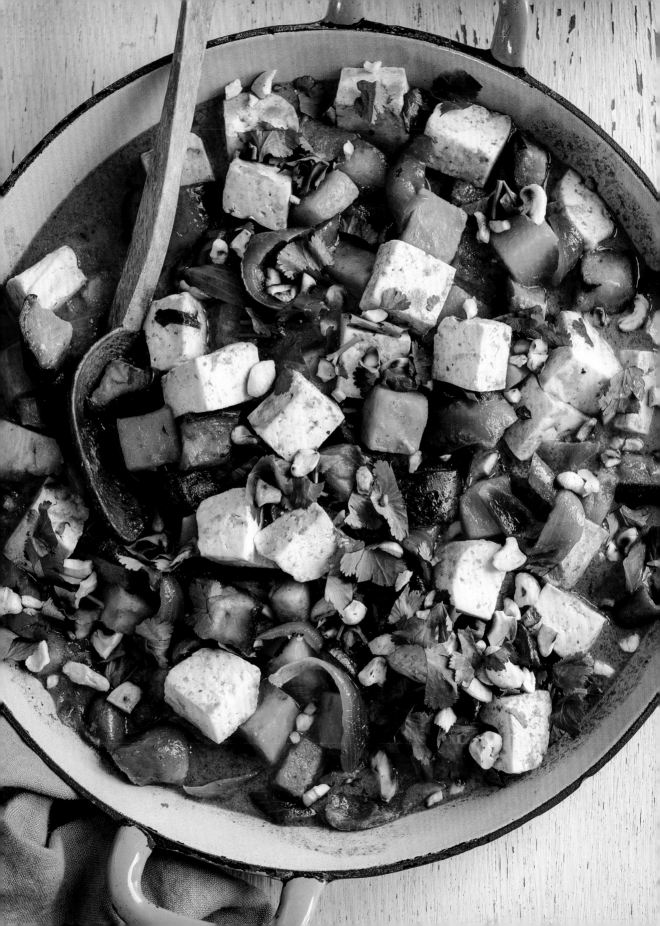

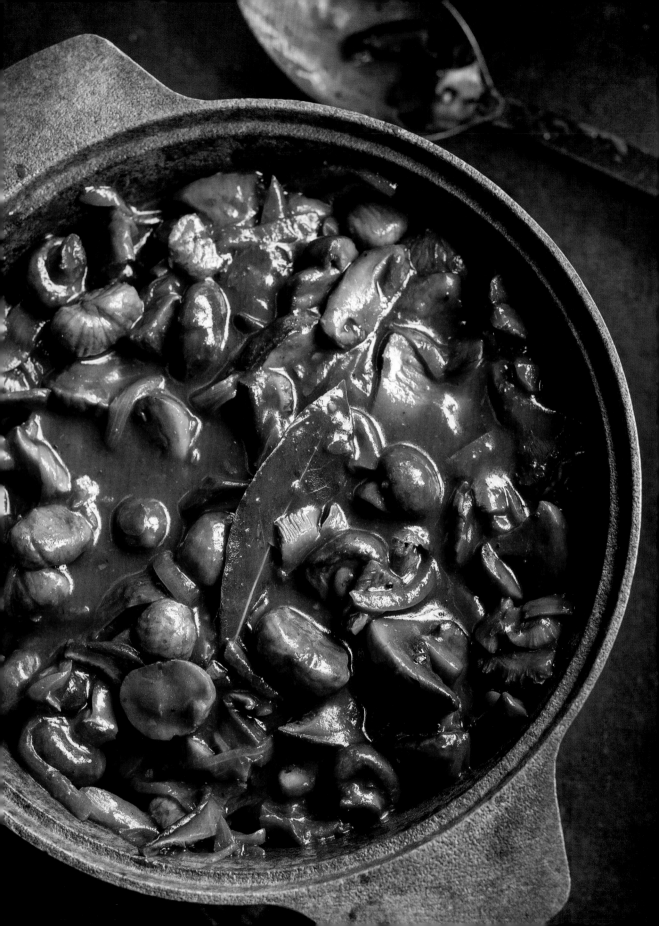

Mushroom and chestnut hot pot

SERVES 4

15g dried mixed mushrooms
2 tbsp olive or rapeseed oil
1 medium onion, peeled
  and thinly sliced
400g mixed mushrooms,
  such as chestnut, shiitake
  and Portobello, sliced
  (or halved if small)
2 garlic cloves, peeled
  and crushed
1 vegetable stock cube
180g cooked and peeled
  chestnuts
100ml red wine (or water)
2 tbsp tomato purée
1 tbsp fresh thyme leaves
  (or 1 tsp dried thyme)
2 bay leaves
4 tsp cornflour

NON-FAST DAYS
Top with roughly chopped
nuts and serve with brown
rice, quinoa or swede
mash (see page 180).

You'll find dried mushrooms with the stock cubes or
in the speciality section of the supermarket. They add
a depth of flavour that makes this dish particularly rich
and delicious. Serve with lots of freshly cooked leafy
greens, kale or shredded Savoy cabbage.

1 Place the dried mushrooms in a measuring jug and cover
with 500ml just-boiled water from a kettle. Stir and leave
to stand for 15 minutes.

2 Heat the oil in a flame-proof casserole and gently fry the
onion and fresh mushrooms for 6–8 minutes, or until the
onion is softened and the mushrooms lightly browned.
Add the garlic and cook for a few seconds more, stirring.

3 Stir in the soaked mushrooms and their liquor, avoiding
any deposits that may have settled at the bottom of the jug.
Add the stock cube and stir in the chestnuts, wine or water,
tomato purée, thyme and bay leaves. Season with sea salt
and ground black pepper. Bring to a simmer, cover the pan
loosely and cook for about 12 minutes, stirring occasionally.

4 Mix the cornflour with 2 tablespoons cold water to form
a thin paste, then stir into the mushroom mixture. Cook for
a further 1–2 minutes, stirring constantly, until the sauce
is thickened and glossy.

COOK'S TIPS

★ If you have time, top the finished dish with 200g peeled
and very thinly sliced celeriac. Cover and bake at 200°C/
fan 180°C/Gas 6 for 20 minutes. Remove the lid and cook
for a further 10 minutes, or until the celeriac is tender
and lightly browned (this will add 14cals per serving).
★ For days when you need more protein and fewer carbs,
you could swap some of the chestnuts for walnuts.

PER SERVING | **232cals** | PROTEIN **8.5g** | FAT **16.5g** | FIBRE **1g** | CARBS **11.5g**

Garlic and herb stuffed mushrooms

SERVES 2

1 tbsp olive oil, plus
    extra for greasing
4 large, flat mushrooms
    (around 250g; such
    as Portobello)
25g wholegrain breadcrumbs
25g ground almonds
10g Parmesan, finely grated
85g medium-fat garlic and
    herb soft cheese
    (such as Philadelphia)
small handful fresh thyme
    leaves (optional)

NON-FAST DAYS
Increase the portion size.
Sprinkle the mushrooms with
a couple of tablespoons of flaked
almonds before baking. Drizzle
with olive oil to serve.

A lovely light lunch or supper. Mushrooms are low
in starchy carbs and have been found to reduce the
risk of cognitive decline. Serve with a generous mixed
leaf salad, drizzled with a little balsamic vinegar.

1 Preheat the oven to 200°C/fan 180°C/Gas 6 and lightly
grease a small baking tray.

2 Twist the stalk out of each mushroom and place the
mushrooms, dark-side up, on the tray.

3 Mix the breadcrumbs with the almonds and Parmesan
in a small bowl and season with sea salt and lots of ground
black pepper. Using half the breadcrumbs, sprinkle some
into each mushroom then dot with small pieces of the
cheese. Top with the remaining breadcrumbs. Drizzle
with the oil and bake for about 12–15 minutes, or until
the crumbs are crisp.

4 Divide the mushrooms between two plates, sprinkle
with fresh thyme, if using, and serve.

COOK'S TIP

★ To make your own crumbs, simply blitz some
wholegrain bread in a food processor. Any extra
can be frozen for another time.

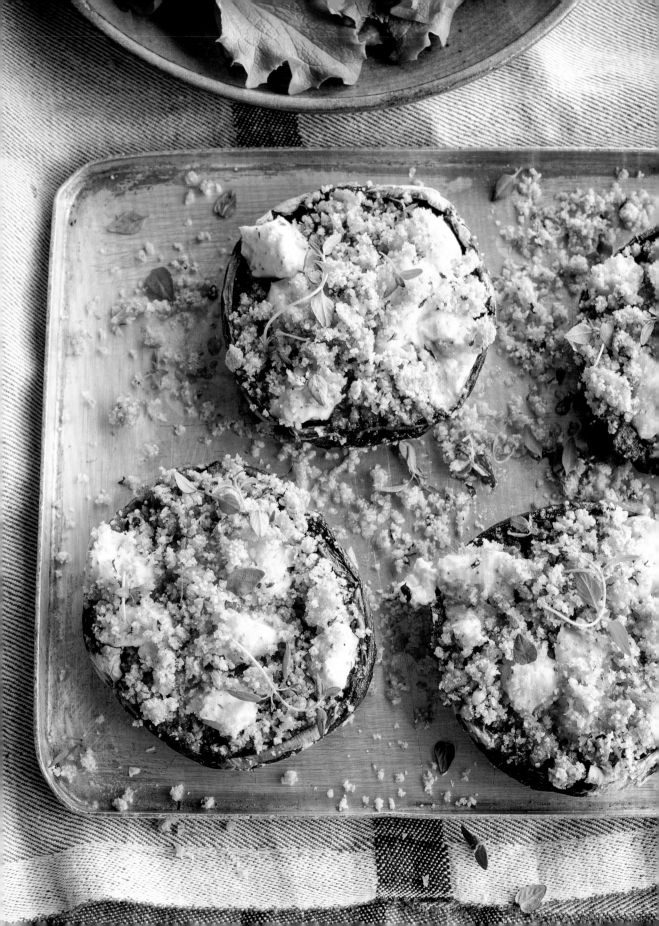

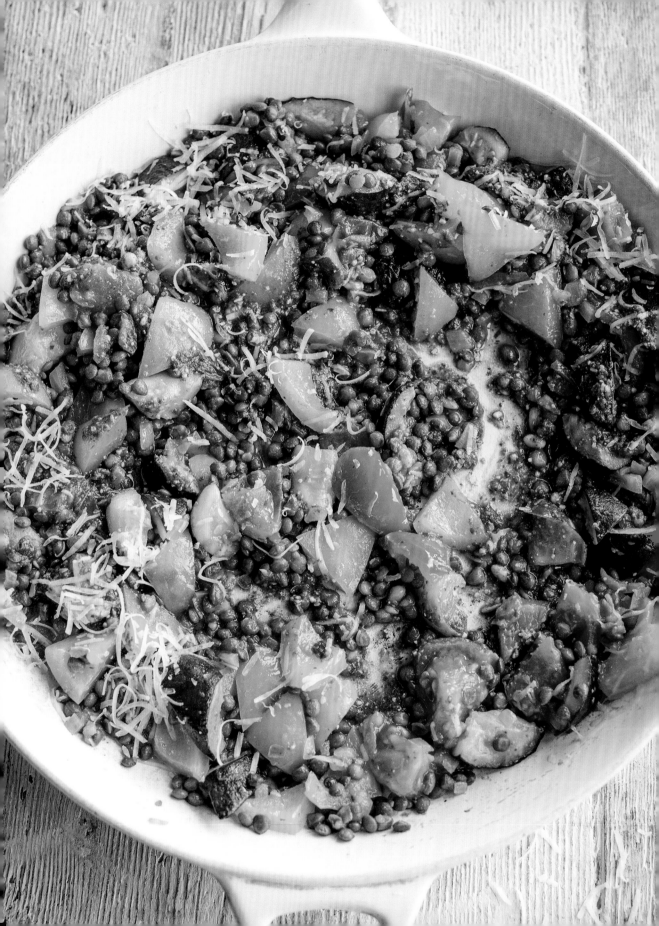

Pesto lentils

1 tbsp olive oil
½ medium onion, peeled
and finely chopped
1 yellow or red pepper,
deseeded and cut into
roughly 2cm chunks
½ medium courgette,
cut into roughly
2cm chunks
2 medium tomatoes,
roughly chopped
1 × 400g can lentils
(any variety), drained
½ vegetable stock cube
2 tbsp basil pesto
20g Parmesan, finely grated

NON-FAST DAYS
Add some warmed wholemeal
pitta bread and extra grated
cheese.

Canned lentils are versatile, cheap and convenient.
Cooked up with fresh veg and pesto, they make a
brilliant quick meal that's packed with fibre and
contains a good protein hit. Serve with a mixed salad.

1 Heat the oil in a large non-stick frying pan and gently
fry the onion, pepper and courgette for 5 minutes, or until
softened and beginning to brown, stirring regularly.

2 Add the tomatoes and cook for 2–3 minutes, or until
the tomatoes are softened, stirring constantly.

3 Add the lentils, crumbled stock cube and 2–3 tablespoons
water. Stir in the pesto and season with lots of ground black
pepper. Cook for 2–3 minutes more, or until the lentils are
hot, stirring constantly.

4 Remove from the heat and sprinkle with the cheese
to serve.

COOK'S TIP

★ For a zingier dish, use fresh basil pesto (found in
tubs in the chilled cabinet at the supermarket). It keeps
for several days in the fridge and can be frozen, too.

PER SERVING | **411cals** | PROTEIN **19g** | FAT **22.5g** | FIBRE **11.5g** | CARBS **28g**

Spicy bean burgers

SERVES 4

1½ tbsp olive oil, plus
    extra for greasing
1 small red onion
    (around 120g), peeled
    and finely chopped
2 garlic cloves, peeled
    and crushed
25g ground almonds
1 medium egg yolk
2 tbsp chipotle or harissa paste
1 × 400g can red kidney beans,
    drained and rinsed
1 × 400g can chickpeas,
    drained and rinsed
75g mixed nuts, roughly
    chopped
25g fresh coriander,
    leaves finely chopped
4 tomatoes, sliced
½ small red onion,
    peeled and finely sliced
100g full-fat live
    Greek yoghurt
lime wedges, to serve

NON-FAST DAYS
Top the burgers with mashed
avocado and toss the salad
in our Simple salad dressing
(see page 241).

These simple burgers are full of flavour. Prepare the
whole batch and you'll have some ready in the freezer
for another day. Serve with a large mixed salad.

1 Preheat the oven to 200°C/fan 180°C/Gas 6. Grease
a baking tray with a little oil.

2 Heat 1 tablespoon of the oil in a large non-stick frying
pan and gently fry the chopped onion for 3–4 minutes,
or until soft, stirring occasionally. Add the garlic and
cook for a few seconds more, stirring.

3 Place the almonds, egg yolk, chipotle or harissa paste,
and roughly half the chickpeas and half the kidney beans
in a food processor and add the fried onion and garlic.
Season well with sea salt and lots of ground black pepper.
Blitz until well combined but not totally smooth.

4 Add the remaining beans, the nuts and fresh coriander
and pulse a few times until combined but with plenty
of texture. Form the mixture into four burgers.

5 Place the burgers on the prepared tray and brush with
the remaining oil. Bake for 25 minutes, or until lightly
browned and hot throughout. Serve one burger per person,
topped with sliced tomato, red onion, the remaining
coriander and spoonfuls of yoghurt, with lime wedges
on the side for squeezing over.

COOK'S TIPS

★ If you can't find chipotle or harissa, use 1 teaspoon each
of ground cumin, ground coriander and hot smoked paprika.
★ You can freeze the cooked burgers wrapped tightly in foil
for up to 3 months. Reheat on a lightly oiled baking tray at
200°C/fan 180°C/Gas 6 from frozen for about 15 minutes,
or until hot throughout.

Curried mince and peas

SERVES 4

2 tbsp olive or rapeseed oil
1 large onion, peeled and
   finely sliced
300g frozen Quorn mince
2 garlic cloves, peeled and
   crushed
20g fresh root ginger,
   peeled and finely chopped
1½–2 tbsp medium curry
   powder or medium
   curry paste
75g dried red split lentils
1 vegetable stock cube
225g frozen spinach
200g frozen peas or a mixture
   of peas and beans

NON-FAST DAYS
Serve with brown basmati
rice and scatter with a handful
of toasted cashew nuts.

A very satisfying, meat-free curry that can be largely cooked from the store cupboard and freezer, and takes less than 30 minutes. Serve with freshly cooked cauliflower rice (see page 242).

1 Heat the oil in a wide-based saucepan or shallow flame-proof casserole and gently fry the onion for 5 minutes, or until softened and lightly browned, stirring regularly.

2 Add the Quorn mince, garlic and ginger and cook for a further 1 minute. Sprinkle in the curry powder, season with sea salt and ground black pepper, and cook for a few seconds more, stirring constantly.

3 Add the lentils, crumble over the stock cube and stir in 800ml water, along with the spinach. Bring the liquid to a simmer. Cover loosely with a lid and cook for 15–20 minutes, stirring regularly, especially towards the end of the cooking time. Simmer uncovered for a little longer, if necessary, to reduce the liquid.

4 Add the peas and cook for 3–5 minutes more, or until the lentils are tender and the peas are hot.

COOK'S TIP

★ The Quorn will continue to absorb the stock as it cools, so you may need to add extra water if reheating. For a non-veggie version, cook 500g turkey mince with 2% fat instead of the Quorn, adding 170cals per serving.

UNDER **400** CALORIES | PER SERVING | **358cals** | PROTEIN **13g** | FAT **19g** | FIBRE **9g** | CARBS **28.5g**

Falafel with harissa vegetables

SERVES 3

1 × 400g can chickpeas,
   drained and rinsed
25g flaked almonds
25g wholemeal flour
2 garlic cloves, peeled
   and crushed
20g fresh coriander,
   leaves roughly chopped,
   plus extra to serve
1 tsp ground cumin
finely grated zest ½ small
   lemon, plus wedges
   for squeezing
1 medium egg yolk
½ tsp flaked sea salt
4 tbsp full-fat live
   Greek yoghurt
1 tbsp extra-virgin olive oil

For the harissa vegetables
1 tbsp harissa paste
1 tbsp extra-virgin olive oil
1 red onion, peeled and
   cut into 12 wedges
2 peppers (1 red and 1 yellow),
   deseeded and cut into
   roughly 2cm chunks
1 courgette, trimmed, halved
   lengthways and cut into
   roughly 2cm chunks

NON-FAST DAYS
Serve with quinoa or bulgur
wheat, or add butternut squash
to the other vegetables.

This versatile, one-pan dish makes a hearty supper
and can be cooled and served as a packed lunch, too.

1 Preheat the oven to 220°C/fan 200°C/Gas 7. Line
a baking tray with non-stick baking paper.

2 Place the chickpeas, almonds, flour, garlic, fresh
coriander, cumin, lemon zest, egg yolk, salt and lots
of ground black pepper in a food processor. Blitz on
the pulse setting to a thick, slightly textured purée.
Form the mixture into 12 balls and flatten slightly.

3 To make the vegetables, mix the harissa paste with
the olive oil in a large bowl and add the onion, peppers
and courgette. Toss well together. Season with sea salt
and lots of freshly ground black pepper then scatter over
the baking tray. Nestle the falafel amongst the vegetables,
drizzle them with the oil and bake for 15 minutes.

4 Remove from the oven, turn the vegetables and falafel
over and return for a further 5 minutes, or until the
vegetables are tender and lightly browned.

5 Mix the yoghurt with around 1 tablespoon cold water
to loosen, stir in some finely chopped fresh coriander,
then drizzle over the vegetables. Serve with lemon
wedges for squeezing.

COOK'S TIPS

★ Each falafel contain 66cals and the vegetables
cooked separately contain 92cals per serving.
★ Use gram flour or gluten-free buckwheat instead
of wholemeal flour for a gluten-free alternative.
★ For extra protein on meat-free days, scatter
25g flaked almonds over the falafel and vegetables
for the last 5 minutes of the cooking time.

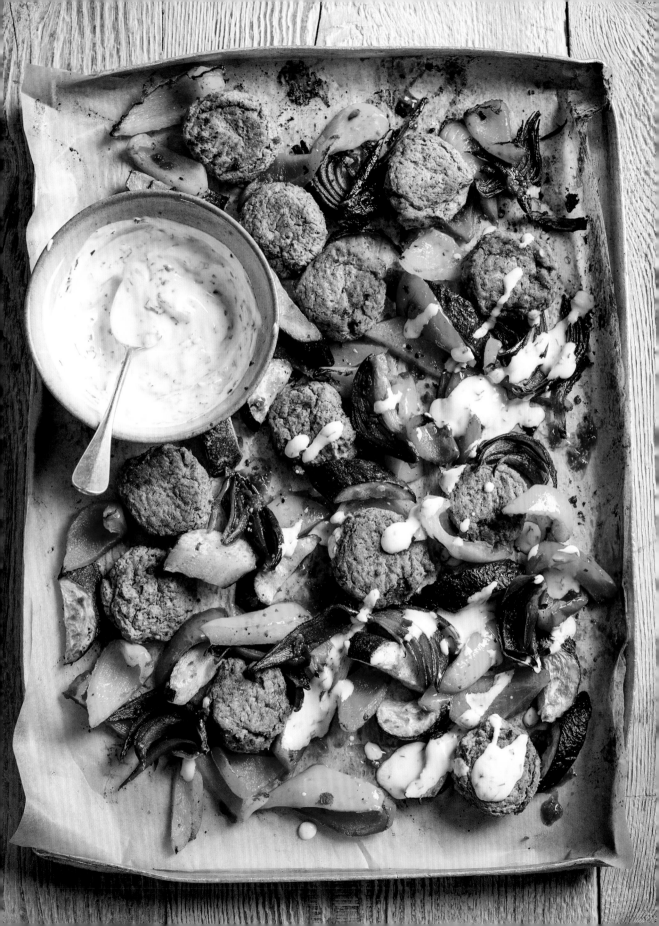

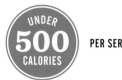

Roasted vegetable pasta with mozzarella

SERVES 2

2 peppers (any colour), deseeded and cut into roughly 2cm chunks

1 medium courgette, trimmed, quartered lengthways and cut into roughly 2cm chunks

1 large red onion, peeled and cut into 12 wedges

2 tbsp olive oil

12 cherry tomatoes, halved

½ tsp crushed dried chilli flakes (to taste)

50g dried bean, pea, lentil or wholewheat penne pasta

50g young spinach leaves

125g mozzarella pearls (mini balls), drained and halved

NON-FAST DAYS

Sprinkle 25g lightly toasted pine nuts or walnuts over the pasta and serve with freshly grated Parmesan and a large mixed salad, tossed with our Simple salad dressing (see page 241).

A comforting, rich dish that's a doddle to prepare. It is best cooked with bean, pea or lentil pasta, which is higher in both protein and fibre and is available in most supermarkets.

1 Preheat the oven to 200°C/fan 180°C/Gas 6.

2 Place the peppers, courgette and onion in a large baking tray. Drizzle with the oil, season with sea salt and lots of ground black pepper and toss together. Roast for 20 minutes.

3 Remove from the oven and turn all the vegetables. Add the tomatoes and sprinkle with the chilli flakes. Cook for a further 10 minutes, or until lightly browned.

4 Meanwhile, half fill a medium saucepan with water and bring to the boil. Add the pasta and stir. Return to the boil and cook for about 10–12 minutes, or until tender, stirring occasionally. Drain the pasta and return to the pan.

5 Add the spinach, roasted vegetables and mozzarella pearls to the pan, toss everything together and season with more ground black pepper. Cook for about 1 minute, stirring until the mozzarella begins to melt and the spinach wilts.

COOK'S TIP

★ To reduce the sugars released when eating a starchy food like pasta by up to 50%, try the cook-cool-cook method (see page 243).

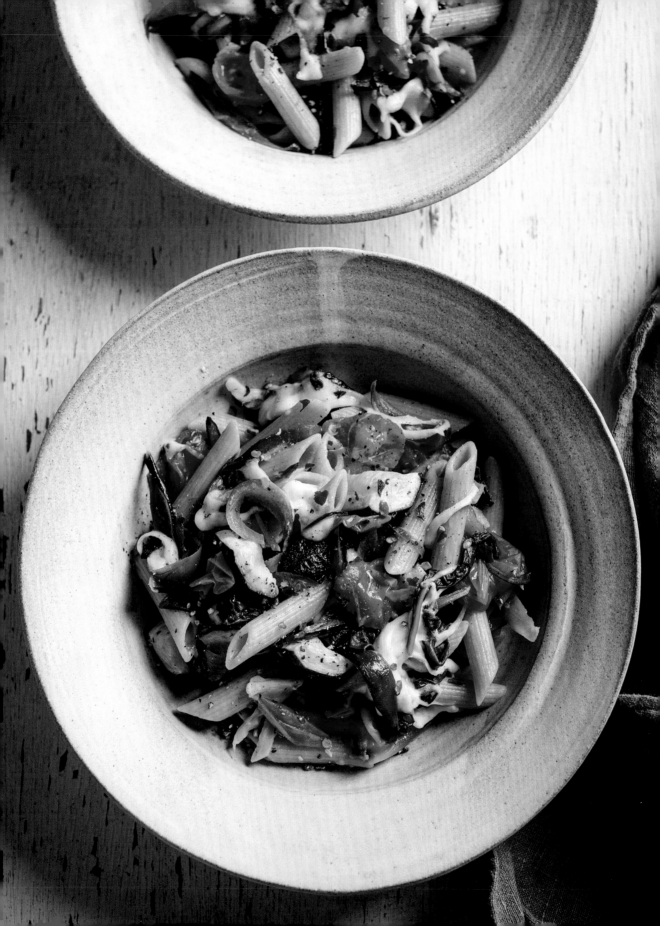

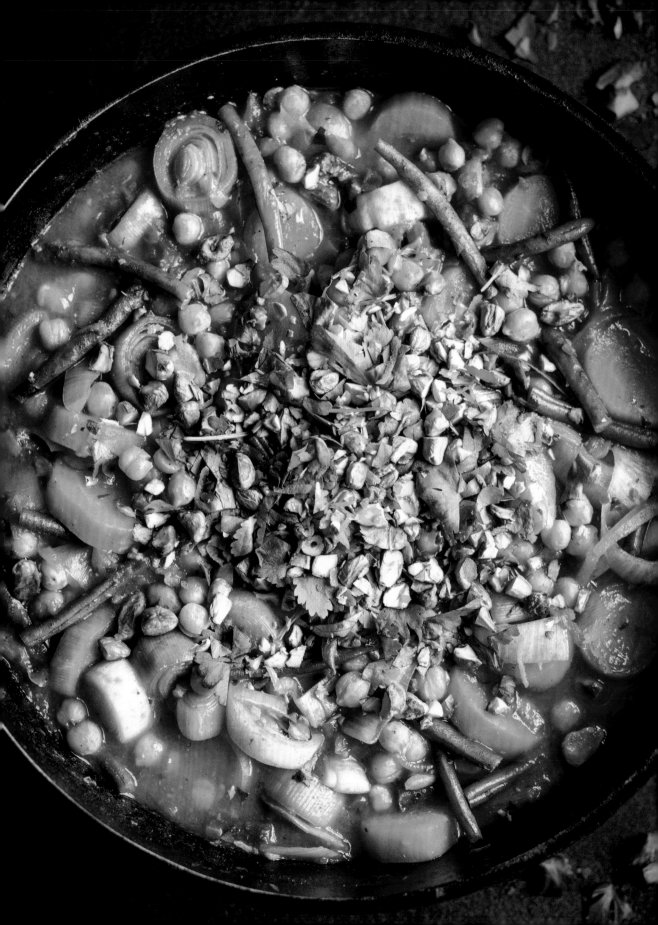

Chickpea and pistachio pot

SERVES 4

1 tbsp olive oil
1 large onion, peeled
   and finely sliced
2 garlic cloves, peeled
   and crushed
2 medium carrots (around
   200g), trimmed and cut
   into roughly 5mm slices
1 × 400g can chopped tomatoes
2 × 400g cans chickpeas,
   drained
2 tbsp harissa paste
1 vegetable stock cube
100g pistachio nuts
1 tsp dried mixed herbs
2 slender leeks, trimmed and
   cut into around 1cm slices
100g fine green beans,
   trimmed and cut in half
20g bunch fresh coriander,
   leaves chopped
finely grated zest ½ orange

NON-FAST DAYS
Increase the portion size
and drizzle liberally with
olive oil. Serve with a small
portion of quinoa or mixed
brown and wild rice.

A golden vegetable stew with a tangy orange and
nut topping. Serve with leafy greens.

1 Heat the oil in a large non-stick saucepan or flame-
proof casserole and gently fry the onion for 5 minutes, or
until softened and lightly browned, stirring occasionally.
Add the garlic and cook for a few seconds more.

2 Stir in the carrots, tomatoes, chickpeas and harissa.
Add 450ml water and crumble over the stock cube.
Tip in half the nuts and the dried herbs, season with
a little sea salt and lots of ground black pepper and stir
well. Bring to a gentle simmer and cook for 10 minutes,
stirring occasionally.

3 Add the sliced leeks, green beans and half the
coriander and cook for 5–10 minutes more, or until
all the vegetables are tender and the sauce has
thickened slightly, stirring regularly.

4 Roughly chop the remaining nuts and mix with the
remaining coriander and the orange zest.

5 Spoon the vegetables into a warm serving dish and
sprinkle the nut mixture over the top.

| PER SERVING | **321cals** | PROTEIN **16g** | FAT **22g** | FIBRE **5g** | CARBS **12g**

Ratatouille and halloumi bake

SERVES 4

2 peppers (1 red and 1 yellow),
    deseeded and cut into
    roughly 2cm chunks
1 medium aubergine
    (around 250g), cut into
    roughly 2cm chunks
1 medium onion, peeled
    and cut into 12 wedges
3 tbsp olive oil
2 garlic cloves, peeled
    and crushed
handful fresh basil leaves
    (around 10g), thinly sliced,
    plus extra to serve
1 × 400g can chopped
    tomatoes with herbs
225g block halloumi cheese,
    cut into 8 slices

NON-FAST DAYS
Add a 400g can of drained
and rinsed cannellini beans
to the ratatouille at the same
time as the tomatoes. Drizzle
the halloumi and vegetables
generously with olive oil
when you serve.

This ratatouille is wonderfully versatile, delicious
served warm or cold. It can be easily reheated in
the microwave, so also makes a handy packed
lunch. Serve with a large leafy salad.

1 Preheat the oven to 220°C/fan 200°C/Gas 7.

2 Place the peppers, aubergine and onion in a bowl, add
2 tablespoons of the olive oil and season with sea salt and
ground black pepper. Toss everything together well then
scatter into a shallow baking dish and bake for 25 minutes.

3 Remove the dish from the oven, turn the vegetables,
then cook for a further 5–10 minutes, or until well
softened and lightly browned.

4 Remove the dish from the oven, stir in the garlic, basil
and tomatoes, arrange the halloumi on top, drizzle with
the remaining oil, season with more ground black pepper
and return to the oven for a further 15 minutes, or until
the halloumi is hot and lightly browned.

5 Scatter with more fresh basil to serve.

COOK'S TIP

★ If you don't have canned tomatoes with added
herbs, simply stir ½ teaspoon dried oregano through
the tomatoes before adding to the vegetables.

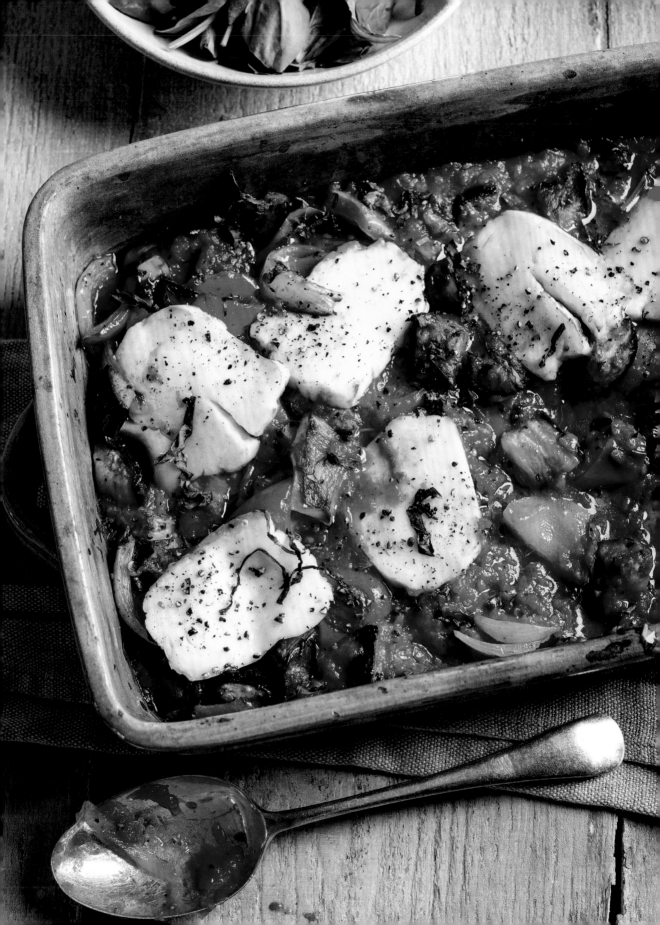

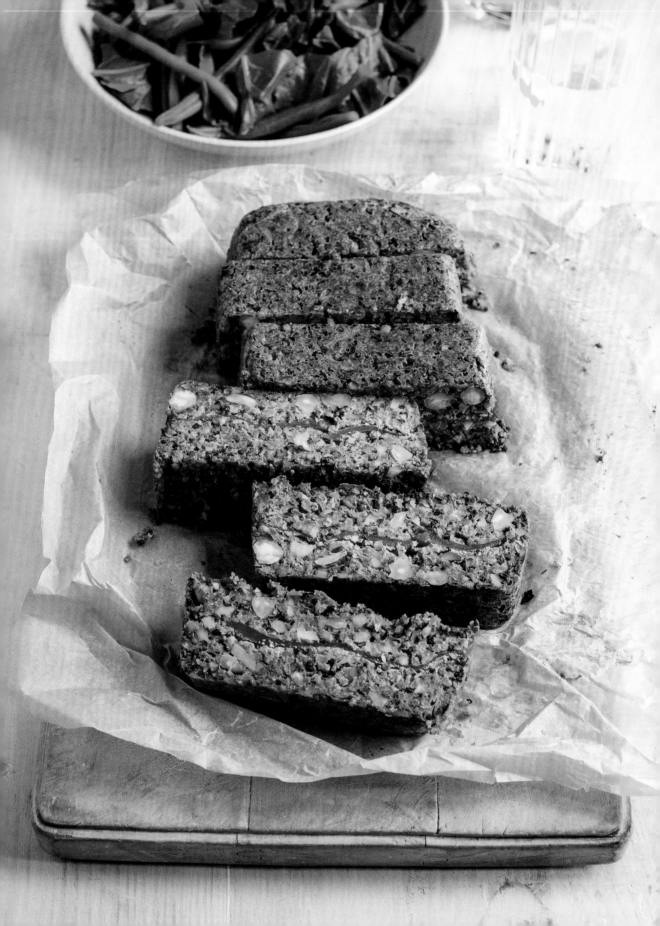

Nut, red pepper and quinoa roast

SERVES 6

1 tbsp olive oil, plus
    extra for greasing
100g quinoa (ideally a mix
    of white, black and red)
1 medium onion, peeled
    and finely chopped
2 garlic cloves, peeled
    and crushed
1 vegetable stock cube
150g mixed nuts,
    roughly chopped
180g cooked and peeled
    chestnuts
2 small carrots, trimmed
    and coarsely grated (about
    100g prepared weight)
2 medium eggs, beaten
finely grated zest 1 lemon
20g fresh parsley,
    leaves finely chopped
150g roasted peppers
    from a jar, drained well

NON-FAST DAYS
Enjoy a larger portion with
a well-dressed salad.

Nut roast has come of age. This one is surprisingly easy to make. Serve warm with vegetables or cold with salad.

1 Preheat the oven to 190°C/fan 170°C/Gas 5. Grease and line the base of a 900g loaf tin with non-stick baking paper.

2 Half fill a pan with water and bring to the boil. Add the quinoa, stir well and return to the boil. Cook for 12–15 minutes, or until tender. Drain very well. (You should end up with 250g cooked quinoa.)

3 Meanwhile, heat the oil in a large non-stick frying pan and gently fry the onion for 5 minutes or until softened. Add the garlic and crumbled stock cube and cook for a few seconds more, squashing the stock cube with a wooden spoon. Tip in the nuts and cook together for 3 minutes, stirring regularly.

4 Place the chestnuts in a large bowl and roughly mash with a potato masher. Add the onion and nut mixture, the cooked quinoa, carrot, beaten eggs, lemon zest and parsley. Season well with sea salt and ground black pepper and mix well.

5 Spoon half the mixture into the tin. Smooth and flatten with the back of a spoon. Arrange the roasted peppers on top, then cover with the remaining nut roast mixture. Press down firmly – this will make it easier to slice when cooked. Cover the tin with foil and bake for 20 minutes.

6 Remove the foil and bake for a further 15 minutes, or until lightly browned and set.

7 Cool in the tin for 5 minutes before turning it out on to a board. Cut into thick slices to serve.

Leek and goat's cheese barley risotto

SERVES 4

1 tbsp olive oil
1 medium onion, peeled
  and finely chopped
2 garlic cloves, peeled
  and crushed
120g pearl barley
1 bay leaf
1 vegetable stock cube
2 medium leeks (around 375g),
  trimmed and cut into
  roughly 5mm slices
50g Parmesan, finely grated
100g goat's cheese, rind
  removed if you prefer
fresh thyme leaves,
  to serve (optional)

5:2

NON-FAST DAYS
Increase the portion size.

The pearl barley adds a wonderful nutty taste and creamy texture to this risotto. Serve with freshly cooked long-stemmed broccoli or kale.

1 Heat the oil in a large non-stick saucepan and gently fry the onion for 3–5 minutes, or until softened and lightly browned, stirring regularly. Add the garlic and cook for a few seconds more.

2 Add the pearl barley and bay leaf. Crumble over the stock cube, add 900ml cold water, cover loosely and bring to the boil.

3 Reduce the heat to a gentle simmer and cook for 40–50 minutes, or until tender, stirring occasionally. Add extra water if the barley absorbs more than expected. It should be nice and saucy.

4 Add the sliced leeks and cook for 5 minutes more, or until tender, then stir in the Parmesan and season to taste with sea salt and lots of ground black pepper.

5 Spoon the risotto on to warmed plates or bowls and crumble the goat's cheese on top. Sprinkle with thyme leaves, if using, to serve.

COOK'S TIP

★ Look out for quick-cook barley, or a mixture of quick-cook barley and other grains; this will only take around 20 minutes to cook but you'll need to reduce the amount of water in the recipe.

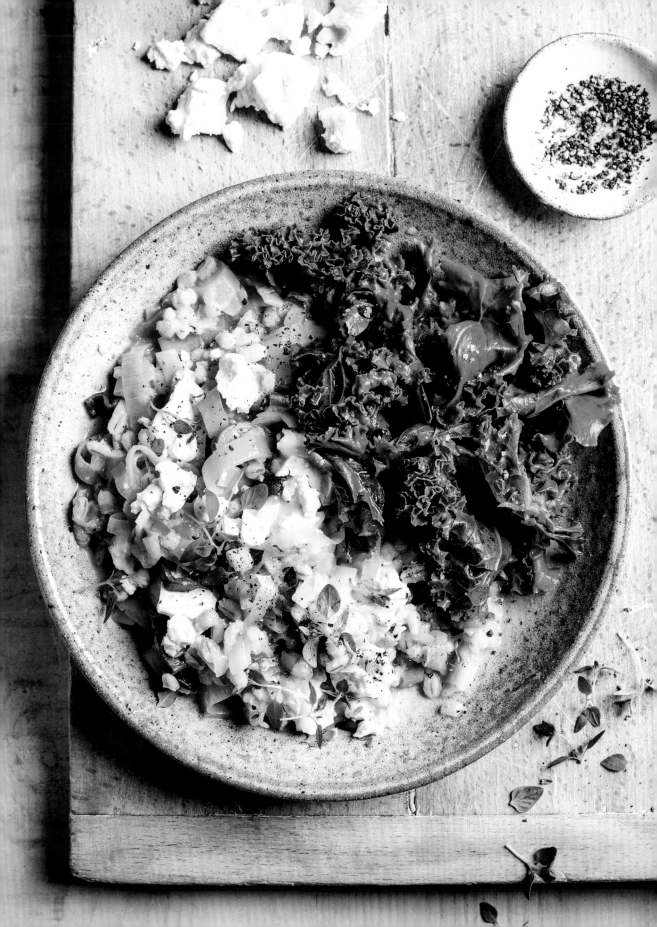

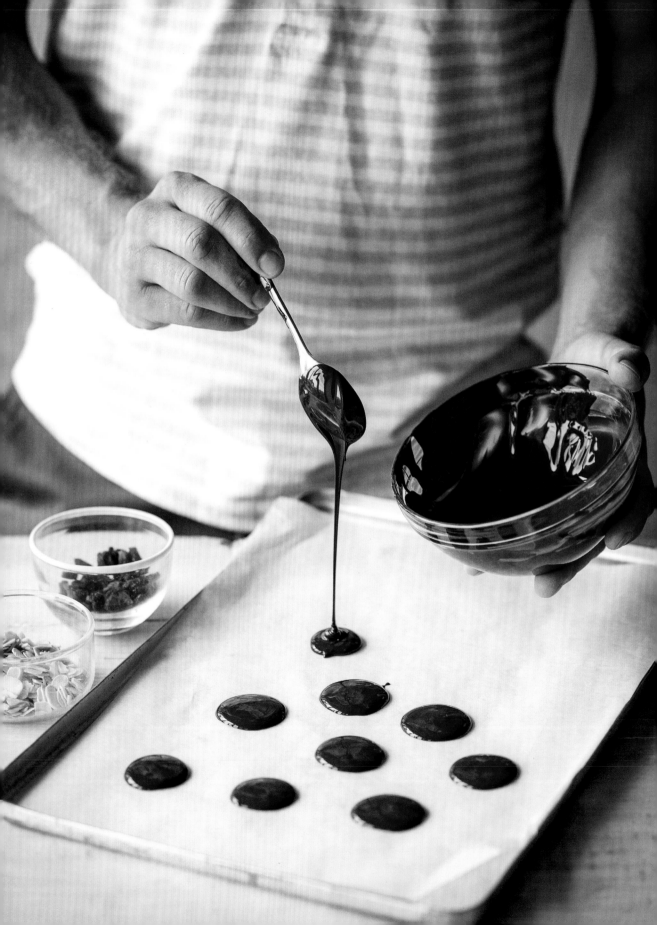

Occasional Treats

In our household, there is no such thing
as willpower – Michael has been spotted
gouging cheesecake straight out of the
freezer with a spoon. The emphasis here is
on the word 'occasional' – these are treats for
enjoyment every now and then, preferably
straight after a meal. We recommend that if
there are leftovers from these recipes, you
divide them into portions and freeze them.
Most of the cakes have a healthy vegetable
base and use ground almonds or wholemeal
flour (instead of white or brown). They are
not light and fluffy like a Victoria sponge,
but we hope you enjoy the firmer texture.
As you retrain your tastebuds, you will
find them increasingly satisfying.

Cinnamon apple crisps

SERVES 2

2 tsp coconut oil
½ tsp ground cinnamon
1 large red-skinned apple
    (around 200g)

5:2

NON-FAST DAYS
Enjoy the crisps dipped
in full-fat yoghurt.

These moreish snacks contain lots of healthy soluble
fibre. Best eaten as a little treat after a meal.

1 Preheat the oven to 130°C/fan 110°C/Gas ½. Line a large
baking tray with non-stick baking paper.

2 Melt the coconut oil in a small saucepan with the
cinnamon over a low heat and set aside.

3 Top, tail and core the apple. Finely slice into discs just
3–4mm thick.

4 Brush the cinnamon oil all over the apple slices, then
place in a single layer on the baking tray. Bake for 1½ hours,
or until very dry and quite crisp.

5 Switch off the oven and leave the apples to dehydrate
further for 2–3 hours.

6 Divide between two people to serve.

COOK'S TIP

★ If you are making these in larger quantities, store any
uneaten apple crisps in a lidded container and eat within
a couple of days.

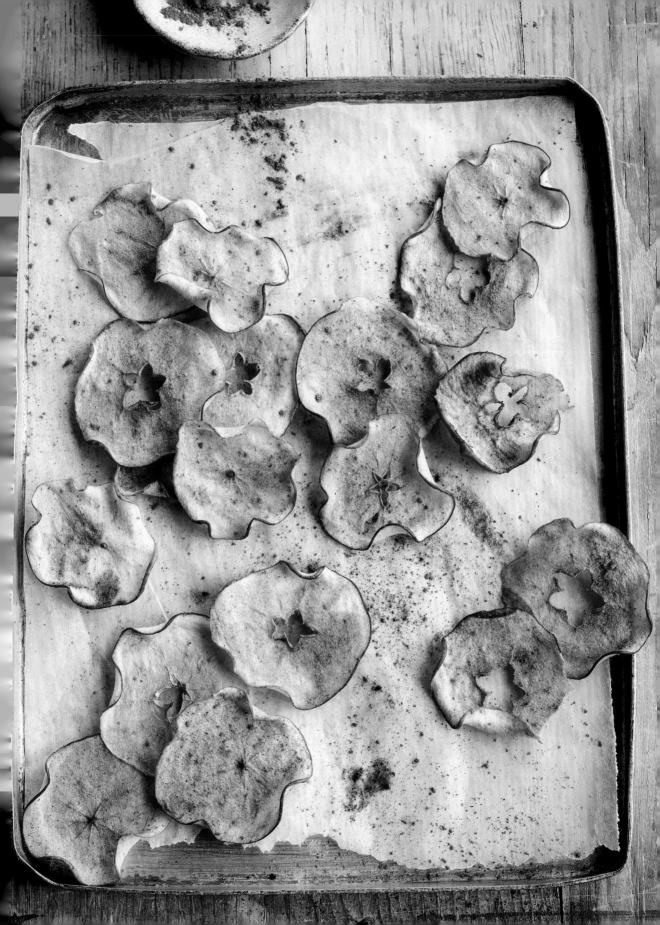

Orange and almond loaf

SERVES 10

2 medium oranges
(each around 150g),
well washed
8 soft pitted dates
4 tbsp olive oil
4 medium eggs
300g ground almonds
1½ tsp baking powder
15g flaked almonds

NON-FAST DAYS
Serve thicker slices or top
with a berry compote and
dollops of crème fraîche
for a gorgeous dessert.

An irresistible, tangy cake. Amazingly, it's cooked
using whole oranges with no need to peel them.
Serve warm in thin slices.

1 Prick each of the oranges 20 times with the tip of a knife
and place in a microwave-proof bowl. Cover with a plate
and microwave on high for 10 minutes, or until very soft.

2 Preheat the oven to 190°C/fan 170°C/Gas 5. Line the base
and sides of a 900g loaf tin with non-stick baking paper.

3 Leave the oranges until cool enough to handle, then cut
in half and remove any seeds. Place the oranges and dates
in a food processor, add the olive oil and eggs and blitz
until thoroughly blended.

4 Add the ground almonds, baking powder and 4 tablespoons
water and blend again to a thick batter. Pour into the
prepared tin, spreading to the sides. Sprinkle with the
flaked almonds and bake for 40–45 minutes, or until
risen, golden brown and firm to the touch.

5 Cool in the tin for 30 minutes, then turn out and cut
into thin slices to serve.

COOK'S TIPS

★ If you don't have a microwave, gently simmer the oranges
in a loosely covered saucepan of water, without pricking,
for 50–60 minutes instead. Top up with water when needed.
★ Keep the loaf wrapped tightly in foil, or save extra slices
in the freezer. You can warm them in the microwave before
eating, if you like.

Ginger and parsnip traybake

SERVES 16
150g coconut oil, plus
   extra for greasing
3 large eggs
50g soft pitted dates, halved
4 tsp ground ginger
1 tsp ground cardamom
   or cinnamon
1 tsp ground nutmeg
1 tsp vanilla extract
250g parsnips (about
   2 medium), peeled
   and coarsely grated
100g wholemeal plain flour
2 tsp baking powder
2 stem ginger balls (around
   30g), drained and cut into
   roughly 1cm chunks

NON-FAST DAYS
Enjoy a larger portion.

This traybake is moist, with delicious bursts
of sweet ginger. And no one would guess that
it contains parsnips!

1 Preheat the oven to 190°C/fan 170°C/Gas 5. Grease and
line the base and sides of a 20cm loose-based square cake
tin with non-stick baking paper.

2 Place the eggs, coconut oil or butter, dates, ground ginger,
cardamom or cinnamon, nutmeg and vanilla in a food
processor and blitz until well combined.

3 Add the parsnips, flour and baking powder and blitz
again on the pulse setting until the mixture comes together
and forms a soft batter.

4 Spoon into the prepared tin, spreading to the sides.
Dot with the chunks of stem ginger and press into the
batter lightly. Bake for 40–45 minutes, or until slightly
risen and golden brown.

5 Leave the cake to cool in the tin for 10 minutes,
then transfer to a wire rack.

6 Cut into 16 squares and serve warm or cold.

COOK'S TIPS

★ There is no need to buy expensive dates for this recipe,
the cheaper ones found in the baking aisle will work fine.
★ Wrap tightly in foil and freeze portions for another day.

| PER SERVING | **207cals** | PROTEIN **3g** | FAT **16g** | FIBRE **3.5g** | CARBS **11g**

Mango and passion fruit pots

SERVES 4

10g unsweetened
   desiccated coconut
2 passion fruit, halved
1 small ripe mango
   (around 300g), peeled,
   stoned and diced
   (see tip below)
finely grated zest ½ small
   lime (optional)
300g coconut milk yoghurt,
   well chilled

NON-FAST DAYS
Toast some mixed nuts with
the coconut in step 1 to make
a richer topping.

A luscious, tropical-tasting dessert.

1 Place the coconut in a small saucepan and toast over
a medium heat for 2–3 minutes, stirring regularly. Leave
to cool.

2 Use a teaspoon to scoop the passion fruit out of the shells
and place in a bowl. Add the mango and lime zest, if using,
and stir well.

3 Divide the mango and passion fruit between four glass
tumblers or dessert dishes, saving a little for decoration.
Top with the yoghurt, then finish with the toasted coconut
and reserved mango mixture.

COOK'S TIPS

★ Make these with full-fat live Greek yoghurt, if you
prefer, for 168cals per pot.

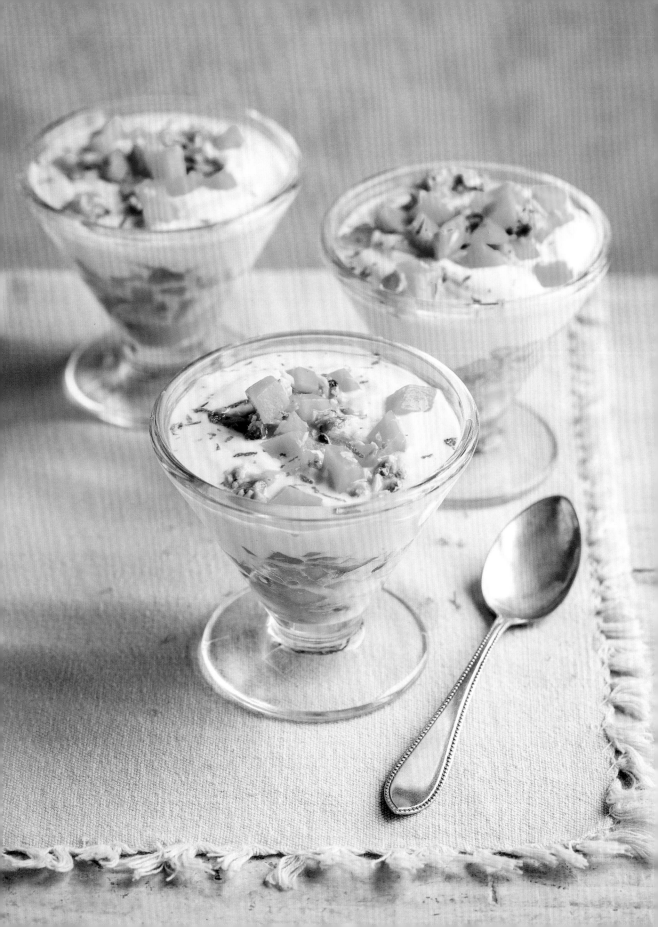

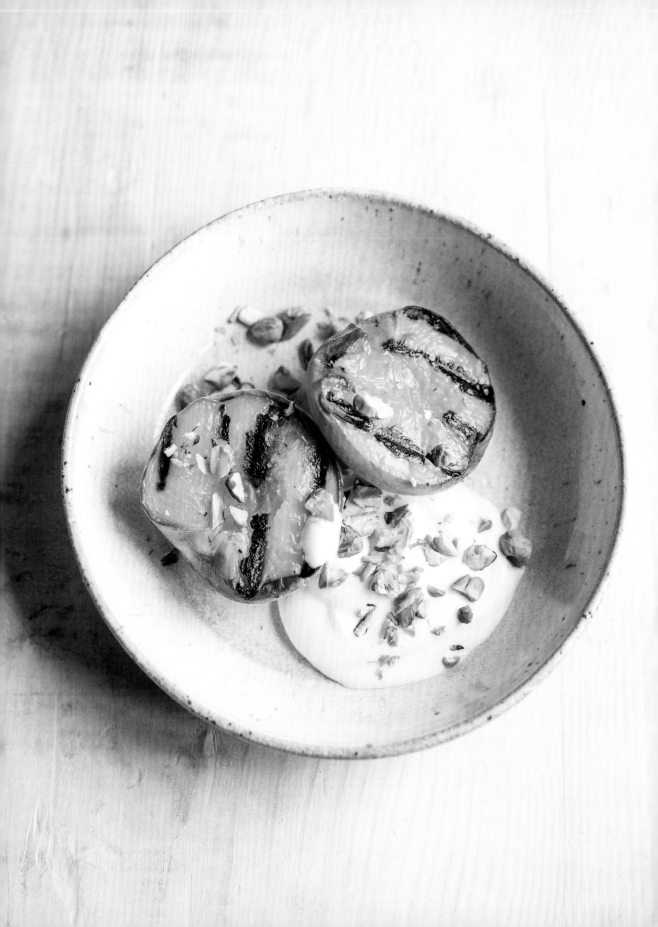

PER SERVING | **130cals** | PROTEIN **6g** | FAT **5.5g** | FIBRE **3g** | CARBS **12g**

Seared peaches with yoghurt and pistachios

SERVES 4

1 tsp olive or rapeseed oil
4 firm but ripe peaches
  or nectarines, halved
  and stoned
150g full-fat live
  Greek yoghurt
25g unsalted pistachio nuts,
  roughly chopped

NON-FAST DAYS
Enjoy a larger portion.

A simple fruit dessert that also works beautifully as a summery breakfast.

1 Place a large griddle pan over a medium–high heat and brush with the oil.

2 Place the peaches on the griddle, cut-side down, and cook, without moving, for about 3 minutes, or until hot and marked with griddle lines.

3 Serve with the yoghurt and a sprinkling of nuts.

COOK'S TIPS

★ If you don't have a griddle pan, grill the peaches instead, or cook in a lightly oiled frying pan.
★ If your peaches don't cut in half easily, cut into slices around the stone instead.

Chocolate mug cake

SERVES 2

1 tbsp coconut oil
4 soft pitted dates (around
    30g), finely chopped
1 medium egg, beaten well
25g ground almonds
7g cocoa powder
    (around 1 tbsp)
¼ tsp baking powder
1 square (around 5g) plain
    dark chocolate (around
    85% cocoa solids)
handful fresh raspberries,
    to serve

You will need a microwave-proof
mug (to hold around 300ml)

NON-FAST DAYS
Serve with a dollop of full-fat
live Greek yoghurt.

Try this for instant gooey-centred chocolate indulgence.

1 Place the coconut oil in the mug and melt in the
microwave on high for a few seconds. Do not allow
to overheat.

2 Add the dates, egg, almonds, cocoa powder, baking
powder and a small pinch of flaked sea salt to the mug and,
using a fork, mix the ingredients until thoroughly combined.
Add an extra 1–2 teaspoons water to loosen the mixture,
if needed.

3 Press the square of chocolate vertically into the top of
the cake batter until submerged and microwave on high
for about 1 minute, or until the cake is risen, firm and
just beginning to shrink from the sides of the mug.

4 Holding the hot mug carefully, turn the cake out on
to a plate and cut in half to reveal the melted chocolate.
Divide between two plates and serve each half with
a handful of fresh raspberries.

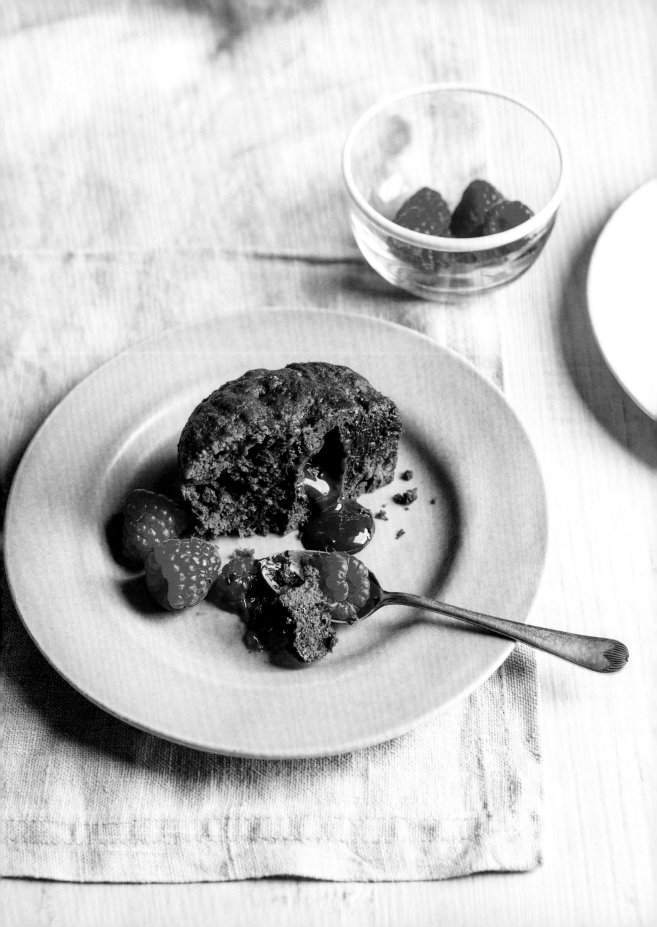

Almond and raisin chocolate pennies

SERVES 20

**100g plain dark chocolate
(around 85% cocoa solids)**
**25g toasted flaked almonds
(see page 18)**
25g raisins

NON-FAST DAYS
Enjoy a larger portion.

It's really worth finding dark chocolate with 85% cocoa solids for these tiny chocolate treats, which are full of beneficial polyphenols that your gut bugs will love. The almonds add some protein and crunch and the raisins bring sweetness and extra fibre.

1 Line a baking tray with non-stick baking paper.

2 Break the chocolate into squares and place in a heat-proof bowl over a pan of gently simmering water, making sure the base of the bowl is not touching the surface of the water. Leave to melt slowly for about 5 minutes, stirring occasionally. Alternatively, microwave on high for 1–2 minutes, or until almost fully melted, then stir. Do not allow to overheat or the chocolate will stiffen or burn.

3 Carefully remove the hot bowl from the pan and, using a teaspoon, pour 20 individual spoonfuls of the melted chocolate on to the tray, spaced well apart.

4 Scatter the almonds and raisins on top of the melted chocolate. Leave to set for a few hours.

5 Using a knife, gently prise the pennies from the baking paper. Place in a lidded container and store for up to a week in a cool place.

COOK'S TIPS

★ If you are toasting your own almonds, leave to cool before sprinkling over the melted chocolate.
★ You can use dried cranberries instead of raisins, if you prefer, but look out for varieties containing less sugar.
★ If you think you might be tempted to eat too many, make half a batch at a time.

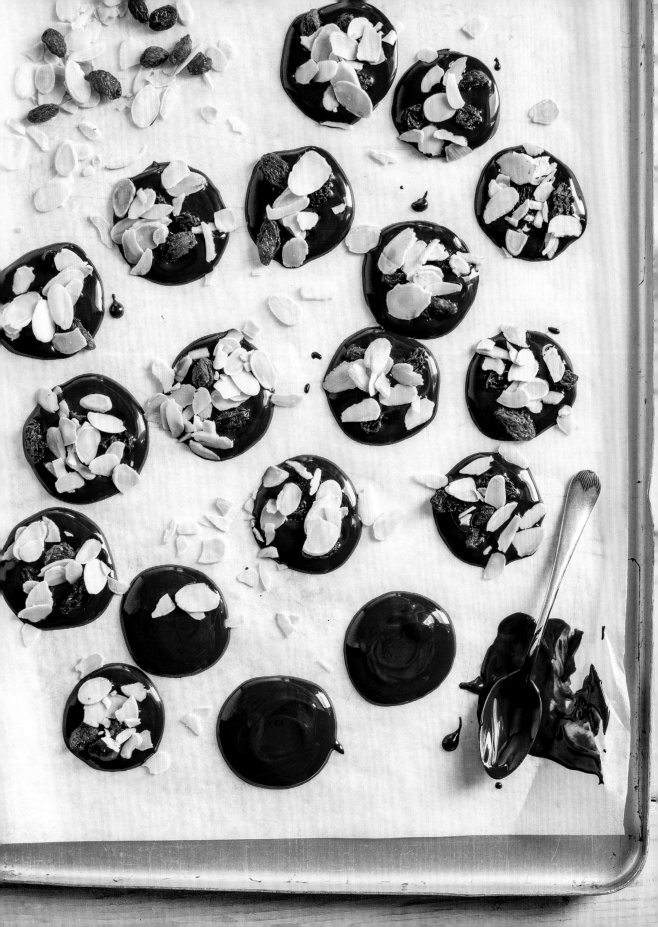

PER SERVING | **170cals** | PROTEIN **3g** | FAT **12.5g** | FIBRE **1.9g** | CARBS **10g**

Byron Bay bars

MAKES 16

125g coconut oil
150g jumbo oats
100g toasted flaked almonds
 (see page 18)
25g flax seeds (linseeds)
75g dried cranberries,
 roughly chopped
2 medium egg whites
2 tsp vanilla extract

NON-FAST DAYS
Enjoy a bar after lunch,
or even for breakfast.

I came across a version of these in a café overlooking Main Beach in Byron Bay, Australia. A lovely, crunchy treat that will give you an energy boost and plenty of fibre. Unlike the shop-bought kind, these bars aren't overly sweet.

1 Preheat the oven to 200°C/fan 180°C/Gas 6. Line the base of a 20cm loose-based square cake tin with non-stick baking paper.

2 Melt the coconut oil in a saucepan over a low heat.

3 Remove from the heat and vigorously stir in the oats, almonds, flax seeds and cranberries and a pinch of sea salt.

4 Whisk the egg whites together until slightly frothy. Add to the oat mixture and mix well.

5 Spoon the mixture into the prepared tin and smooth the surface with the back of a spoon, pressing down well to compress all the ingredients. Bake for 15–18 minutes, or until lightly browned.

6 Leave to cool in the tin for at least 1 hour before cutting into slim bars.

COOK'S TIP

★ Freeze the bars in an airtight container, layering with non-stick baking paper. Thaw individual bars for about 1 hour.

Fudgy chocolate bars

SERVES 20

150g mixed nuts,
  roughly chopped
150g soft pitted prunes,
  quartered
150g ready-to-eat dried
  apricots, quartered
25g cocoa powder
50g coconut oil (not melted)

NON-FAST DAYS
Serve with a dollop of full-fat
yoghurt or crème fraîche.

**Really rich no-bake bars that make a great alternative
to sugary confectionery and contain plenty of fibre.
An occasional indulgence, best eaten after a meal.**

1 Line a 900g loaf tin with cling film, leaving plenty
overhanging the sides.

2 Place the nuts in a food processor and blitz until
finely chopped but not ground. Tip into a bowl. Add the
prunes and apricots to the food processor and blend
to a thick paste.

3 Return the nuts to the food processor and add the cocoa
powder and coconut oil. Blend until the mixture forms
a rough ball.

4 Spoon into the prepared tin, spreading to the sides. Cover
the top of the chocolate mixture with the overhanging cling
film. Place in the freezer for 1 hour, or until solid.

5 Remove from the freezer, unwrap and place on a board.
Cut into 20 × roughly 1cm bars. Store in a lidded container,
layering with sheets of baking paper so the bars don't stick
together. Keep in the fridge for up to 2 weeks, or in the
freezer for 2 months.

COOK'S TIP

★ If you have a large food processor, you can add all the
ingredients at the same time instead of in batches.

PER SERVING | **123cals** | PROTEIN **4.5g** | FAT **8g** | FIBRE **2.5g** | CARBS **7g**

Strawberry and vanilla yoghurt

SERVES 4

250g fresh strawberries,
hulled and halved
300g full-fat live
Greek yoghurt
½ tsp vanilla extract

5:2

NON-FAST DAYS
Enjoy with an extra portion
of strawberries.

A super-easy yoghurt that makes a great dessert
or breakfast. Strawberries have a natural sweetness
but are surprisingly low in sugar.

1 Place the strawberries in a mixing bowl and mash
to crush the berries and release their juices.

2 Mix the yoghurt and vanilla in a separate bowl,
then lightly fold in the strawberries.

3 Divide between small dishes or glasses and
keep chilled.

COOK'S TIP

★ You can use frozen strawberries or mixed berries
for this recipe, just make sure they are well thawed
and drained before you mash them.

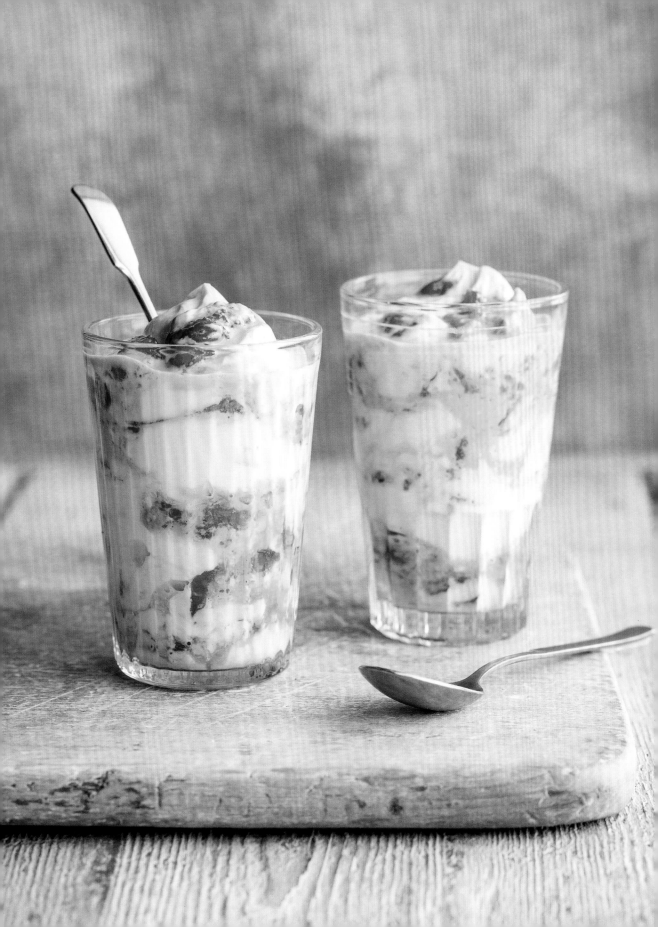

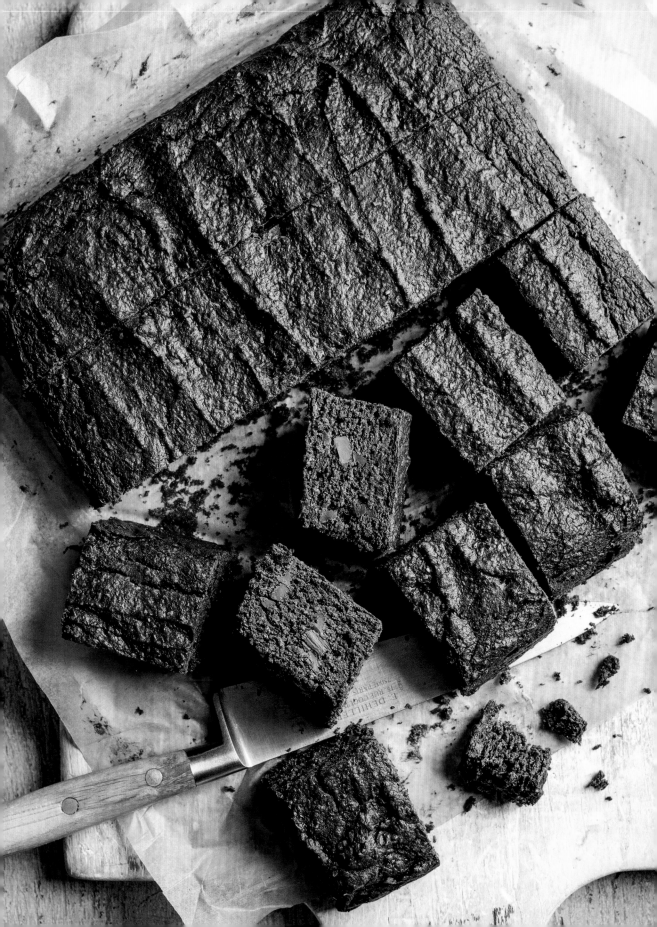

Chocolate beetroot brownies

SERVES 20

100g coconut oil, plus
    extra for greasing
275g cooked beetroot, drained
    and cut into small chunks
3 large eggs
60g cocoa powder
100g soft pitted dates
100g wholemeal
    self-raising flour
1 tsp ground cinnamon
1 tsp bicarbonate of soda
75g plain dark chocolate
    (around 85% cocoa solids),
    roughly chopped

NON-FAST DAYS
To add a bit of crunch and
extra protein, throw in 150g
roughly chopped pecans with
the chocolate. Serve after a
meal with a handful of berries,
a dollop of full-fat yoghurt or
crème fraîche. (You can reheat
in the microwave for a few
seconds first, if you like.)

Challenge anyone to identify the main ingredient!

1 Preheat the oven to 200°C/fan 180°C/Gas 6. Grease and
line the base and sides of a 20cm loose-based square cake
tin with non-stick baking paper.

2 Place the beetroot, eggs, cocoa powder, dates and coconut
oil in a food processor and blend until thoroughly combined.
You can also blend the ingredients together in a bowl using
a stick blender.

3 Add the flour, cinnamon, a pinch of sea salt and the
bicarbonate of soda and blend until well combined. Add
an extra tablespoon water to loosen the mixture, if needed.
Stir in the chocolate, then spoon into the prepared tin,
spreading to the sides. Bake for about 20 minutes, or
until risen and just firm to the touch.

4 Cool in the tin for 10 minutes, then turn out and
cut into squares to serve.

COOK'S TIPS

★ If you use a pack of ready-cooked beetroot from the
supermarket, make sure it doesn't contain vinegar or
spices! Otherwise, you can cook them yourself – wash
the beetroot, place in a pan of water, bring to the boil
and cook for 40–45 minutes, or until tender, then peel.
★ Freeze leftover brownies in a lidded container,
wrapped in foil.

PER SERVING | **178cals** | PROTEIN **6.5g** | FAT **4g** | FIBRE **4g** | CARBS **27.5g**

Seeded wholemeal bread

SERVES 12

7g sachet dried
   fast-action yeast
425g strong wholemeal
   bread flour, plus 1 tbsp
   extra for kneading
100g mixed seeds
2 tbsp skimmed milk powder
1 tbsp soft light brown sugar
1½ tsp fine sea salt
1 tbsp olive oil, plus
   extra for greasing

A lovely loaf and slightly chewy. Store leftover slices in the freezer. Ideal for a bread maker.

1 Mix the yeast, flour, seeds, milk powder, sugar and salt in a large bowl and make a well in the centre.

2 Fill a jug with 150ml just-boiled water from a kettle and top up with 200ml cold water to give a total of 350ml lukewarm water. Add the oil and pour into the flour mixture. Using a large spoon, stir to combine into a rough ball.

3 Turn out on to a lightly floured surface and knead for 5 minutes. The dough will be very sticky so add a little flour to the surface if necessary. Place in a lightly oiled bowl, cover with cling film and leave to rise in a warm place for 1½–2 hours, or until almost doubled in size.

4 Gather the dough and form gently into a ball. Line a baking tray with baking paper and place the dough on top. Form into a roughly 18cm round. Score three times with a sharp knife, cover loosely in oiled cling film and leave to prove for 1–1½ hours, or until well risen.

5 Preheat the oven to 220°C/fan 200°C/Gas 7. Remove the cling film and bake for 25 minutes, or until golden brown. The base should sound hollow when tapped. Cool on a wire rack. Serve in thin slices – one serving should be around 65g.

COOK'S TIPS

★ This bread can be made very successfully in a bread maker on the wholewheat setting.
★ To make a homemade crispbread, cut the 1–2-day-old loaf into very thin slices, each around 15g, and place on a baking tray in a preheated oven at 170°C/fan 150°C/Gas 3. Bake for about 20 minutes or until crisp and completely dry. Store in an airtight container.

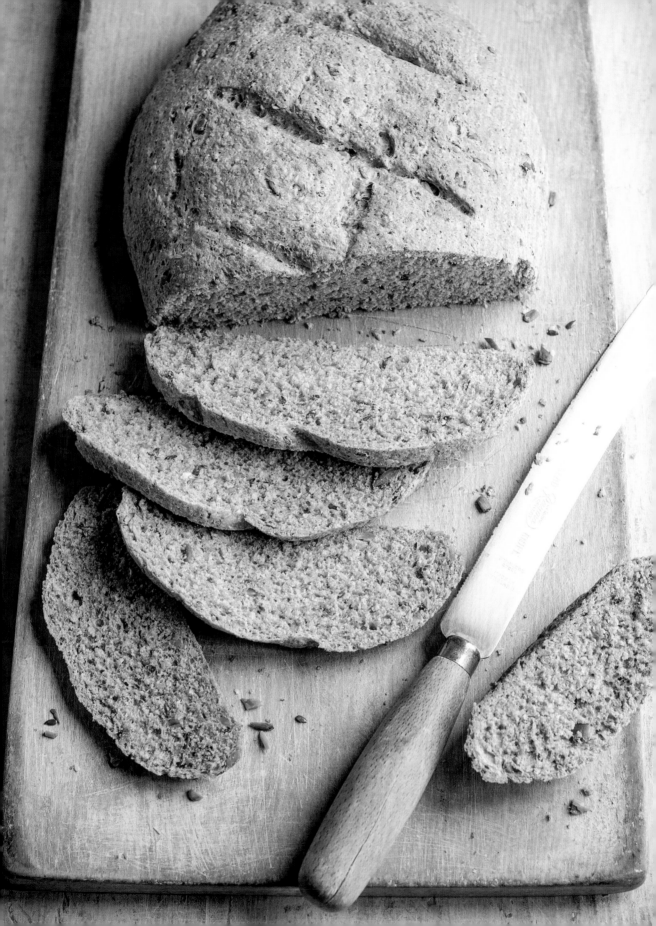

Your Fast 800 toolkit

Easy ways to maintain your protein intake

Maintaining an adequate protein intake is important when you are fasting. Protein is needed to build and repair tissues such as bones, muscle and cartilage, as well as to make enzymes and hormones, and to support the functioning of a healthy immune system. It also makes meals more filling. We recommend eating around 45–60g protein daily. It is harder for vegetarians to achieve this on 800 calories, so they may need to increase to around 900cals a day to ensure they get enough.

Here are some simple calorie-counted suggestions to help you adapt a dish, whether you are on an 800cals day or a non-fast day, either to increase the protein content or make a meal more satiating. They are particularly useful if you haven't got time to cook a full recipe and you're just starting with a plate of non-starchy veg, or you want something to scatter on a soup or salad.

Meat & fish
- 75g cooked chicken breast (115cals)
- 1 tbsp diced chorizo, about 10g (29cals)
- 1 tbsp chopped fried bacon, about 7g (23cals)
- 75g frozen cooked prawns, defrosted (59cals)
- 45g tuna, canned in oil (85cals)
- 3 drained anchovies in oil (17cals)

Dairy & egg
- 1 tbsp grated cheese, about 10g (41cals)
- 30g Cheddar – about matchbox-sized (124cals)
- 30g halloumi, sliced, lightly fried in 1 tsp olive oil for 4–5 mins (145cals)
- 1 tbsp full-fat live Greek yoghurt, about 40g (37cals)
- 15g full-fat feta (54cals)
- 10g Parmesan (42cals)
- 1 medium egg (78cals)

Vegetarian
- Handful of nuts, around 10g, e.g. walnuts, almonds, hazelnuts (185cals)
- 2 tsp sesame seeds, about 10g (60cals)
- 15g almonds (95cals)
- 100g tofu (73cals)
- 80g cooked edamame beans (85cals)
- 15g mixed seeds (55cals)
- 100g cooked puy lentils (143cals)

Ways to jazz up your greens and non-starchy veg

Greens and non-starchy vegetables are such an important part of the Fast 800 that we encourage you to eat these freely, filling half of your plate with each meal. Steam, boil or microwave them, and then try some of these ideas to make them taste even better. We list minimal-calorie options, for when you are at your 800cals limit, and low-calorie options, for when you've got some calories going spare.

Examples of greens and non-starchy veg: cabbage, spring greens, chard, kale, pak choi, cavolo nero and spinach; as well as green beans, mange tout, sliced courgette, broccoli or peppers. And salad leaves of all colours – the more colourful the better.

Minimal-calorie ways to add flavour:
- Flaked sea salt and black pepper
- A pinch of crushed dried chilli flakes
- A little crushed garlic
- ½ tbsp dark soy sauce
- A squeeze of lemon or lime, e.g. on cabbage, broccoli or cauliflower
- ½ tbsp live cider vinegar or balsamic vinegar, e.g. on spinach or cavolo nero

Low-calorie ways to add flavour:
- 1 tsp butter – good on any veg (25cals)
- 1 tsp olive oil – good on any veg (27cals)
- 1 tsp hoisin sauce, e.g. on wilted spinach or cabbage (12cals)
- 1 tsp sesame or nigella seeds, e.g. on fine green beans or cabbage (32cals)
- 1 tsp grated Parmesan scattered on top, e.g. steamed broccoli (8cals)
- ½ garlic clove and ½ tbsp olive oil (plus 1 tsp soy sauce) – good for stir-frying cabbage, mange tout, broccoli or chard (52cals)

SALAD DRESSINGS

These calorie-counted dressings will enhance any plate of leafy greens. Do also feel free to mix and match the salads in Chapter 3 with their dressings to suit you.
- Minted yoghurt dressing – page 71
- Cider vinegar dressing – page 74
- Mustard dressing – page 76
- Yoghurt dressing with herbs – page 78
- Soy and lime dressing – page 80
- Lime dressing – page 84
- Creamy garlicky yoghurt dressing – page 86
- Lemon mayo, non-fast day – page 116
- Balsamic dressing – page 178
- Simple olive oil and lemon juice dressing – page 72
- **Simple salad dressing**
  Place 1 tsp Dijon mustard, 1 tbsp balsamic vinegar and 5 tbsp extra-virgin olive oil in a screw-top jar and season with a good pinch of sea salt and lots of ground black pepper. Fasten the lid and shake really well. Adjust the seasoning to taste. Serve 1 tablespoon of the dressing per person for 102cals. Use within 5 days.

OTHER SIDES AND SAUCES

If you have the calories spare, these sides and sauces will boost any dish.
- Homemade coleslaw – page 87
- Tomato sauce – page 177 (63cals per serving)
- Moroccan-style tomato sauce – page 177 (92cals per serving)
- Quick pickled cucumber – page 146 (insignificant added calories)
- Satay sauce – page 153 (154cals per serving)
- Minty yoghurt raitha – page 106
- Sautéed mushrooms – fry 40g mushrooms in 1 tsp olive oil (63cals)
- Olives – 5 pitted olives in brine (25cals)

How to embrace healthier carbs

The Fast 800 is all about ditching the starchy white stuff – white bread, pasta, potatoes and rice – and embracing complex carbs instead, like wholegrains, beans and lentils, which contain important nutrients and are an excellent source of fibre.

WHOLEGRAINS

We recommend you cook these in larger quantities and freeze them in portions. Crumble in half a stock cube during cooking for added flavour. Beans and lentils are a particularly good source of protein for vegetarians and are good for gut bacteria too. Add around 2 heaped tablespoons on a fasting day, depending on what calories you have to spare, or 3 tablespoons on a non-fast day.

- 1 tbsp cooked brown rice, around 15g (21cals)

- 1 tbsp cooked quinoa, around 15g (18cals)

- 1 tbsp cooked bulgur wheat, around 15g (13cals)

- 1 tbsp cooked puy lentils, around 15g (18cals)

- 1 tbsp cooked pearl barley, around 15g (19cals)

LOW-CARB SWAPS

For alternatives to starchy foods, you might like to try some of these. Cauliflower makes an excellent swap as it's very low in calories and high in nutrients. It's also remarkably flexible. We love it.

- **Cauliflower rice** (200g) 34cals (see page 129) Hold a small cauliflower at the stalk end and coarsely grate in sort, sharp movements in a downward direction only to create tiny shavings of cauliflower resembling grains of rice. You can also do this in a food processor but don't let the pieces get too small or they will turn to a paste. Either add the raw cauliflower rice to a stir-fry, or steam or sauté for 3–4 minutes to cook. You can do this in the microwave – place in a microwave-proof bowl and cook on high for 2–3 minutes. The rice should retain a bit of bite, like al-dente pasta. Stir in some chopped parsley or coriander, or squeeze over some fresh lemon juice for added flavour.

- **Cauliflower mash** 84cals (see step 1 on page 160)

- **Courgetti spaghetti** (100g) 20kcals (see page 168) Allow 1 courgette per person. Use the large noodle attachment of a spiralizer or a potato peeler to make the courgetti. Steam, boil or microwave the courgetti for about 1 minute, or until al dente. If you have the spare calories, heat a drizzle of olive oil in a frying pan and cook the courgetti for about 1 minute, or until softening, and season with a pinch of salt and plenty of black pepper.

- **Squash mash** 55cals (see steps 2 and 4 on page 166)

- **Swede mash** 71cals (see step 4 on page 180)

- **Pea and broccoli mash** 161cals (see step 3 on page 128)

- **Celeriac chips** 64cals (see step 2 on page 182)

- **Cabbage linguini** (100g) 27cals Use ¼ Savoy cabbage for 2 people. Remove the core, finely slice the cabbage then steam for 4–5 minutes or in the microwave for less. You want it to be al dente.

- **Konjak 'zero' noodles or spaghetti** (shiritaki). Originally from Japan, these contain remarkably few calories and plenty of fibre. They are available in most large supermarkets.

Resistant starch or the cook-cool-cook approach

Many people find it hard to give up all starchy carbs. Fortunately, there is some new research which suggests that the way you cook these foods can reduce the amount of sugar you absorb.

The cook-cool-cook technique is a way of converting some of the starch in foods such as potatoes, pasta and rice into 'resistant starch', which resists digestion and instead behaves more like fibre. Your microbiome loves it and you can eat these foods with less of a blood sugar spike. Remember that this method only converts some of the starch, though, so you still need to eat it in moderation!

To do this, first cook your pasta, rice or potatoes as you would normally. Then cool them, ideally for 12 hours in the fridge. When you heat them up fully again, you enhance the effect, converting some of the simple starch into non-digestible resistant starch.

Tips for using the cook-cool-cook approach to convert to resistant starch

- Always choose brown versions of rice or pasta in the first place.

- Store portions in the freezer, so you have them ready to defrost and heat up. You can also scatter pre-cooked grains on a salad or eat them with a meal. Pre-cooked rice is ideal in a stir-fry.

- For your non-fast days, you can make delicious pasta dishes or bakes in advance and reheat portions as needed.

- Keep brown bread in the freezer (which is also a great way to avoid the temptation to finish the loaf) and stick it straight in the toaster.

PREP TIPS AND WHERE TO FIND THEM

- How to toast nuts or seeds – toast nuts in a dry frying pan over a low heat for around 2 minutes, stirring frequently until lightly browned in places. Seeds need less time.
- How to spiralise veg – see opposite
- How to prepare an avocado – see tip on page 40
- How to poach an egg – see recipe on page 34
- Homemade chicken stock – see tip on page 65
- Quick pickled veg – see recipe on page 147

Good hydration with minimal calories

Regular fluid intake is vital on a fast day to keep your energy levels up. Aim to drink an extra 1–1.5 litres of calorie-free fluids, mainly as water. It is best to avoid drinks with sweeteners as they can upset the good bugs in your gut; they are also likely to maintain your sweet tooth as they are many times sweeter than sugar. If you drink a lot of artificially sweetened drinks, you may need to reduce them over a matter of days or even weeks to avoid withdrawal and cravings. If you must use a sweetener, Stevia is probably best.

Do try some of these lovely ways to add flavour without significant calories. These drinks can be had any time and won't interfere with fat-burning.

COLD REFRESHING DRINKS

We love tap water and drink it straight from the tap, or filtered. If you find you are inclined to forget to increase your fluid intake, try keeping a jug or bottles in the kitchen or at work – ones that need to be finished by the end of the day. Or carry a bottle with you.

If you are not a fan of plain water, here's how you can make it more enticing:

- Keep bottles of water in the fridge as it tastes better cold.

- For more flavour, include a few berries or some fresh herbs, like mint, rosemary or thyme. Or you might add a squeeze of fresh lemon or lime, and drop a twist of the peel into the bottle. A slice or two of cucumber or courgette looks and tastes refreshing. Make up some fruit or herbal tea, cool it and keep it in the fridge.

HOT COMFORTING DRINKS

Try to avoid putting milk in your tea or coffee between meals as this adds calories and interferes with fat-burning – although, added straight after a meal, a dash of milk is fine. For interest, try sipping fruit teas to distract your taste buds. Or have herbal infusions, adding a handful of fresh herbs, such as mint, thyme or sage, to boiled water.

For a feisty flavoured ginger tea: Finely slice about 1cm of an unpeeled ginger root, drop it in a mug and fill with boiling water. Squeeze in some lemon juice to taste, and allow to steep for about 5 minutes. Ginger is a source of magnesium, which helps bone formation. It has been found to reduce blood pressure and can reduce inflammation – as well as getting you through a fasting day...

EXTRA SUPPORT

It can make a real difference to have a partner, family member or diet buddy doing the diet with you in some way. Try to enlist friends, family, colleagues, and anyone interested to help keep you motivated. For more information, see our website www.thefast800.com where you can also access the Fast 800 Online Programme to help you stay on track and integrate the Fast 800 into your life. Time limited 20% discount code offer for the online programme: F800SUPPORT20

Wishing you all the best on your Fast 800 journey!

MEAL PLANNERS

These meal plans are intended to inspire and give you a start but they are also flexible: feel free to repeat a day so you don't have to cook two days in a row, use up your leftovers and swap in different recipes from the book that you like the look of – whatever best suits your life and work. Just keep an eye on the nutritional information on the recipe pages to make sure you are getting adequate protein (ideally more than 45g) and keeping starchy carbs and sugar lowish (try not to go over 75g carbs on most days and ideally keep it just below 50g).

Remember, the 800cals a day figure is just a guide: going over by 40–50cals here and there is not going to make a significant difference to the rate of weight loss. Some days your total calories may be closer to 900cals, but this will level out over the week.

You will see that in the meat-free plans the daily calorie total tends to be higher – this is to ensure adequate daily protein is included.

If you have calories to spare, you might want to choose a dressing for your salad or try some of the other ideas on page 241 to jazz up your non-starchy vegetables. On some days, you might want to include a portion of hard fruit, such as an apple or pear, or a handful of berries to take you just over the 800cals. On others, we have fallen far enough below the 800cals for you to have an occasional treat (see pages 220–239).

The important thing, if you want to encourage fat-burning, is to stick to a lowish-carb diet, avoid snacking between meals, and ideally add in some Time Restricted Eating (see page 11 for more on this).

RECIPES FOR ONE OR MANY

Lots of the recipes in this book make two or four servings, on the basis that in most cases one portion can be stored in the fridge and eaten in the following day or two; or it can be frozen. If, however, you are cooking for larger numbers, and/or including people who are not restricting calories, simply increase their portion sizes as per the non-fast day suggestions. Non-fasters can also add extra complex carbs, such as brown rice, with plenty of added extra-virgin olive oil, flavourings or dressing as appropriate.

With meat/fish 2 meals a day

Week 1

DAY 1
- Leek and salmon quiche in a dish (507cals) (see page 124)
- Simple steak and salad (346cals) (see page 178)

853cals

DAY 2
- Overnight oats (351cals) (see page 22)
- Chicken wrapped in Parma ham (321cals) (see page 143)

672cals

DAY 3
- Chicken Caesar-ish salad (300cals) (see page 78)
- Mediterranean fish bake (384cals) (see page 117)

684cals

DAY 4
- Salmon salad bowl (542cals) (see page 80)
- Peppered pork stir-fry (276cals) (see page 165)

818cals

DAY 5
- Poached eggs with mushrooms and spinach (241cals) (see page 34)
- Beef stroganoff (392cals) (see page 181) – serve with 40g portion brown rice (147cals)

780cals

DAY 6
- Shakshuka (312cals) (see page 42)
- One-pot roast chicken (460cals) (see page 140)

772cals

DAY 7
- Poached eggs with mushrooms and spinach (241cals) (see page 34)
- Chicken tikka masala (427cals) (see page 148) – serve with 40g portion brown rice (147cals)

815cals

Week 2

DAY 8
- Smashed avocado on toast (289cals) (see page 40)
- Baked salmon with pea and broccoli mash (440cals) (see page 128)

729cals

DAY 9
- Instant porridge in a cup (399cals) (see page 23)
- Chicken, pepper and chorizo bake (421cals) (see page 150)

820cals

DAY 10
- Smoked salmon omelette (339cals) (see page 36) – add a dressing to your salad (see page 241)
- Spicy bean chilli (346cals) (see page 192)

685cals

DAY 11
- Tuna Niçoise salad (362cals) (see page 86)
- Chicken goujons with Parmesan crumb (399cals) (see page 139)

761cals

DAY 12
- Edamame and tuna salad (408cals) (see page 83)
- Easy chicken tagine (447cals) (see page 144)

855cals

DAY 13
- Pear and cinnamon porridge (267cals) (see page 18)
- Lamb chops with crushed minted peas and feta (542cals) (see page 172)

809cals

DAY 14
- Chicken, bacon and avocado salad (495cals) (see page 76)
- Mussels with creamy tarragon sauce (381cals) (see page 132)

876cals

Meat-free 2 meals a day

Week 1

DAY 1
- Smashed avocado on toast (289cals) (see page 40) – serve topped with 1 poached medium egg (78cals) per person
- Spicy bean burgers (411cals) (see page 204) – serve with celeriac chips (64cals) (see page 182)
842cals

DAY 2
- Quinoa, broccoli and asparagus salad (362cals) (see page 71)
- Dan's veggie Bolognese (207cals) (see page 194) – serve with 40g wholewheat pasta (130cals) and 10g grated Parmesan (42cals) per person
741cals

DAY 3
- Hummus, carrot and spinach low-carb wrap (see page 95) – serve a double portion (2 wraps or 1 large wrap) per person (468cals)
- Roasted vegetable pasta with mozzarella (460cals) (see page 208)
928cals

DAY 4
- Gut-friendly chicory with blue cheese and walnuts (335cals) (see page 74) – add 1 sliced hard-boiled egg (78cals) per person
- Chickpea and pistachio pot (397cals) (see page 211)
810cals

DAY 5
- Nut, red pepper and quinoa roast (330cals) (see page 215) – add a dressing to your salad (see page 241)
- Spicy bean chilli (346cals) (see page 192) – add a dressing to your salad (see page 241)
676cals

DAY 6
- Mushrooms on toasted sourdough (297cals) (see page 39) – serve topped with 1 poached medium egg (78cals) per person
- Spicy bean burgers (411cals) (see page 204) – serve with celeriac chips (64cals) (see page 182)
850cals

DAY 7
- Poached eggs with mushrooms and spinach (241cals) (see page 34)
- Ratatouille and halloumi bake (see page 212) – serve an extra-large portion by dividing the bake into three instead of four (428cals)
669cals

Week 2

DAY 8
- Cowboy baked beans (309cals) (see page 46) – serve with 20g grated Cheddar (82cals)
- Dan's veggie Bolognese (207cals) (see page 194) – serve with cabbage linguini (see page 242), 10g grated Parmesan (42cals) and add a dressing to your salad (see page 241)
640cals

DAY 9
- Shakshuka (312cals) (see page 42)
- Falafel with harissa vegetables (358cals) (see page 206) – serve sprinkled with an extra 10g flaked almonds (63cals) per person and add a dressing to your salad (see page 241)
733cals

DAY 10
- Goat's cheese frittata (294cals) (see page 100)
- Spicy bean chilli (346cals) (see page 192) – add a dressing to your salad (see page 241)
640cals

DAY 11
- Blueberry pancakes (284cals) (see page 25) – serve with 2 tablespoons full-fat live Greek yoghurt (74cals) and 10g flaked toasted almonds (63cals) per person
- Curried mince and peas (292cals) (see page 205)
713cals

DAY 12
- Fast falafel, hummus and beetroot salad (395cals) (see page 105)
- Mushroom and vegetable biryani (322cals) (see page 195) – serve with Minty yoghurt raitha (59cals) (see page 106)
776cals

DAY 13
- Boiled eggs with long-stemmed soldiers (216cals) (see page 38)
- Creamy cashew and tofu curry (598cals) (see page 196) – serve with 25g wholewheat noodles (82cals) per person
896cals

DAY 14
- Goat's cheese frittata (294cals) (see page 100) – add a dressing to your salad (see page 241)
- Chickpea and pistachio pot (397cals) (see page 211)
691cals

With meat/fish 3 meals a day

Week 1

DAY 1
- Boiled eggs with long-stemmed soldiers (216cals) (see page 38)
- Mediterranean tuna lettuce wrap (196cals) (see page 90)
- Easy chicken tagine (447cals) (see page 144)
859cals

DAY 2
- Overnight oats (351cals) (see page 22)
- Broccoli and blue cheese soup (158cals) (see page 56)
- Swedish spicy carrot with cod (279cals) (see page 118)
788cals

DAY 3
- Nutty banana shake (214cals) (see page 51)
- Mike's peppered mackerel paté (298cals) (see page 97)
- Spicy bean chilli (346cals) (see page 192)
858cals

DAY 4
- Bacon, broccoli, tomato and mushroom fry-up (144cals) (see page 45)
- Bean soup with kale and pesto (249cals) (see page 54)
- Pan-fried pork with apple and leek (355cals) (see page 163)
748cals

DAY 5
- Warm berry compote with yoghurt (190cals) (see page 26)
- Creamy mushroom soup (68cals) (see page 64)
- Chicken tikka masala (427cals) (see page 148)
685cals

DAY 6
- Shakshuka (312cals) (see page 42)
- Pesto bean salad lettuce wrap (308cals) (see page 91)
- Turkey fajitas (195cals) (see page 154)
815cals

DAY 7
- Blueberry pancakes (284cals) (see page 25)
- Prawn mayo lettuce wrap (143cals) (see page 91)
- One-pot roast chicken (460cals) (see page 140)
887cals

Week 2

DAY 8
- Poached eggs with mushrooms and spinach (241cals) (see page 34)
- Clear chicken and pea soup (280cals) (see page 65)
- Ginger and chilli baked fish (233cals) (see page 120)
754cals

DAY 9
- Instant porridge in a cup (399cals) (see page 23)
- Smoked salmon and cream cheese low-carb wrap (200cals) (see page 94)
- Meatballs in tomato sauce (272cals) (see page 177)
871cals

DAY 10
- Smashed avocado on toast (289cals) (see page 40)
- Curried chicken and lentil soup (223cals) (see page 66)
- Ratatouille and halloumi bake (321cals) (see page 212)
833cals

DAY 11
- Chocolate granola (274cals) (see page 20)
- Mediterranean tuna lettuce wrap (196cals) (see page 90)
- Pan-fried fish with lemon and parsley (368cals) (see page 114)
838cals

DAY 12
- Overnight oats (351cals) (see page 22)
- Broccoli and blue cheese soup (158cals) (see page 56)
- Simple chicken casserole (303cals) (see page 142)
812cals

DAY 13
- Iced berry shake (190cals) (see page 50)
- Speedy pizza (221cals) (see page 189) – add a dressing to your salad (see page 241)
- Classic burger with celeriac chips (259cals) (see page 182) – add a dressing to your salad (see page 241)
670cals

DAY 14
- Bacon, broccoli, tomato and mushroom fry-up (144cals) (see page 45)
- Almost instant noodle soup (210cals) (see page 62)
- Lamb chops with crushed minted peas and feta (542cals) (see page 172)
896cals

Meat-free 3 meals a day

Week 1

DAY 1
- Poached eggs with mushrooms and spinach (241cals) (see page 34)
- Pesto bean salad lettuce wrap (308cals) (see page 91)
- Falafel with harissa vegetables (358cals) (see page 206)

907cals

DAY 2
- Nutty banana shake (214cals) (see page 51)
- Speedy pizza (221cals) (see page 189)
- Spicy bean chilli (346cals) (see page 192)

781cals

DAY 3
- Boiled eggs with long-stemmed soldiers (216cals) (see page 38)
- Asparagus, pea and mint frittata muffins (154cals) (see page 99)
- Spicy bean burgers (411cals) (see page 204) – serve with celeriac chips (64cals) (see page 182)

845cals

DAY 4
- Overnight oats (351cals) (see page 22)
- Goat's cheese frittata (294cals) (see page 100)
- Dan's veggie Bolognese (207cals) (see page 194)

852cals

DAY 5
- Boiled eggs with long-stemmed soldiers (216cals) (see page 38)
- Leek and goat's cheese barley risotto (306cals) (see page 216)
- Mushroom and chestnut hot pot (212cals) (see page 199) – serve sprinkled with 25g toasted nuts over each portion (150cals)

884cals

DAY 6
- Warm berry compote with yoghurt (190cals) (see page 26) – serve sprinkled with 20g toasted flaked almonds (126cals) per person
- Broccoli and blue cheese soup (158cals) (see page 56) – add 50g frozen edamame (53cals) per serving to the soup after blending and heat thoroughly
- Chickpea and pistachio pot (397cals) (see page 211)

924cals

DAY 7
- Boiled eggs with long-stemmed soldiers (216cals) (see page 38)
- Falafel with harissa vegetables (358cals) (see page 206) – add a dressing to your salad (see page 241)
- Spicy bean chilli (346cals) (see page 192)

920cals

Week 2

DAY 8
- Smashed avocado on toast (289cals) (see page 40) – serve topped with 1 poached medium egg (78cals) per person
- Bean soup with kale and pesto (249cals) (see page 54)
- Ratatouille and halloumi bake (321cals) (see page 212)

937cals

DAY 9
- Banana and pecan muffin (322cals) (see page 29)
- Goat's cheese frittata (294cals) (see page 100)
- Mushroom and chestnut hot pot (212cals) (see page 199) – serve sprinkled with 25g toasted nuts (150cals) per person

978cals

DAY 10
- Poached eggs with mushrooms and spinach (241cals) (see page 34)
- Quinoa, broccoli and asparagus salad (362cals) (see page 71)
- Dan's veggie Bolognese (207cals) (see page 194)

810cals

DAY 11
- Strawberry and vanilla yoghurt (123cals) (see page 234)
- Gut-friendly chicory with blue cheese and walnuts (335cals) (see page 74) – serve with 1 sliced hard-boiled egg (78cals) per person
- Chickpea and pistachio pot (397cals) (see page 211)

933cals

DAY 12
- Chocolate and strawberry shake (195cals) (see page 51)
- Garlic and herb stuffed mushrooms (232cals) (see page 200) – serve with 80g cooked edamame beans (85cals) per person
- Spicy bean burgers (411cals) (see page 204)

923cals

DAY 13
- Poached eggs with mushrooms and spinach (241cals) (see page 34)
- Spiced bean and spinach soup (200cals) (see page 59)
- Leek and goat's cheese barley risotto (306cals) (see page 216)

747cals

DAY 14
- Strawberry and vanilla yoghurt (123cals) (see page 234)
- Hummus, carrot and spinach low-carb wrap (see page 95) – serve a double portion (2 wraps or 1 large wrap) per person (468cals)
- Roasted vegetable pasta with mozzarella (see page 208)– reduce the mozzarella to 75g and save 64cals per person (396cals)

987cals

Index of recipes by calories

Fast 800 Stores

Our store cupboard list is intended as a helpful guide. We have included ingredients which come up regularly in our recipes in bold – all of these should be easy to find in a good-sized supermarket – but please don't feel you have to go out and buy every item on the list. Adapt your store cupboard to suit you and feel free to substitute with similar alternatives.

OILS & VINEGARS

Olive oil
Coconut oil
Rapeseed oil
Live cider vinegar
Balsamic vinegar

HERBS & SPICES

Dried oregano
Dried mixed herbs
Flaked sea salt (such as Maldon)
Ground cumin
Ground coriander
Ground turmeric
Smoked paprika
Medium curry powder
Black peppercorns for grinding
Crushed dried chilli flakes

NUTS AND SEEDS

Mixed nuts (such as almonds, pecans, hazelnuts, Brazil nuts and walnuts)
Ground almonds
Flaked almonds
Cashew nuts
Walnuts
Pecans
Mixed seeds (such as sunflower, pumpkin, sesame and flax)

DRIED FOODS

Oats (jumbo and/or rolled)
Canned chopped tomatoes
Quinoa
Stock cubes
Wholewheat flour
Baking powder
Brown rice
Brown basmati rice
Wild rice
Wholewheat pasta and noodles
Red lentils

CANNED & BOTTLED

Chickpeas
Beans – cannellini, borlotti, butterbeans, **haricot,** red kidney beans
Canned tuna
Anchovies
Coconut milk

FLAVOURINGS, SAUCES & PASTES

Harissa paste
Thai red or green curry paste
Medium curry paste
Dark soy sauce
Tomato purée

FRIDGE

Eggs
Full-fat live Greek yoghurt
Cheese – mature Cheddar, goat's cheese, Parmesan, feta
Leafy greens and salad
Lemons
Limes
Garlic
Ginger
Fresh parsley
Fresh coriander
Hummus
Smoked mackerel
Chicken breasts
Cooked chicken
Chorizo
Bacon

FREEZER

Edamame (soya beans)
Peas
Spinach
Frozen mixed vegetables
Prawns
Frozen berries

SWEET THINGS

Soft pitted dates
Maple syrup
Honey
Vanilla extract
Plain 85% chocolate

Index